Manufacturing Victims

Manufacturing Victims

WHAT THE PSYCHOLOGY INDUSTRY IS DOING TO PEOPLE

TANA DINEEN

With a Foreword by
DAVID SMAIL

CONSTABLE · LONDON

First published in Great Britain 1999
by Constable and Company Limited
3 The Lanchesters
162 Fulham Palace Road
London W6 9ER
A previous edition of this book was published in Canada by
Robert Davies Multimedia Publishing Inc. 1996
Second, revised edition, 1998

ISBN 0 094 79790 0

Set in Monotype Bembo 11½pt by
Rowland Phototypesetting Ltd

A CIP catalogue record for this book
is available from the British Library

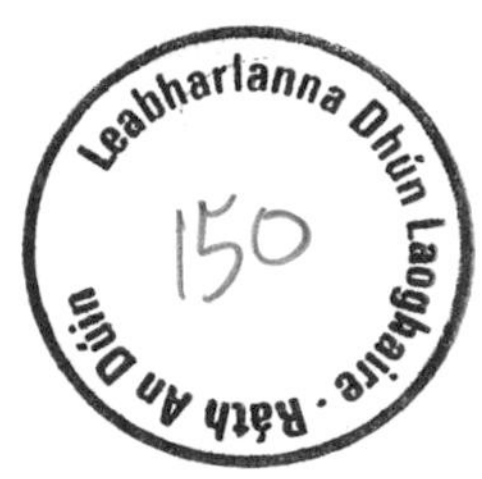

For the old woman with a scar across her face who shouted:
'Never call me a victim!'

Contents

Acknowledgements

I am indebted to those people who, throughout my life, have encouraged me to ask questions and to challenge assumptions.

I consider myself fortunate that my first psychology course was taught by Donald Hebb, a distinguished scholar whose natural curiosity, openness and humility I will never forget. I must acknowledge, as well, the influence of Aldred Neufeldt who, as my research adviser in graduate school, repeatedly demonstrated how concepts such as ethics, integrity and tolerance could be brought to life.

When the North American edition of *Manufacturing Victims* was first released, Aldred was one of the friends from the past to resurface and express support. Sam Keen, a former editor of the popular magazine *Psychology Today*, was another. Sam got back in touch saying that the book was long overdue and that he hoped it would force people to take 'a hard look at the sins of the profession'. I heard also from Theodore Roszak, the historian whose term 'counterculture' came to describe the hippies of the sixties. He recalled our spirited conversations about contemporary society and welcomed my book as 'an antidote for our society's spreading addiction to toxic therapy'.

In addition to these old friends who resurfaced, new ones have emerged. After reading an early draft of the manuscript, Alan Gold, a prominent Canadian lawyer, offered enthusiastic words of support. His constructive criticism and the wealth of material he freely provided helped the book to take shape.

Once it was finished, others appeared, expressing solidarity. Among them were Robyn Dawes and Elizabeth Loftus, two extremely courageous US colleagues who had for a very long time been openly challenging the authority of modern-day psychology. Almost immediately both became tremendous ongoing sources of solid information, stimulating ideas and genuine encouragement.

I would like to thank, as well, Leonard Bickman, whose research embodies the best of what psychology can be and whose voice is one of those that deserve to be heard above the chorus of entrepreneurial 'experts' who avoid the questions and persist in selling 'the answers'. It is good to know that there are such voices in the wilderness and that there are, among my colleagues, people whom I can truly respect.

Finally, I want to express my appreciation to my husband, George Matheson, who accepts me for the sceptic that I am, takes my questions seriously and who is ultimately both my most brutal critic and my most supportive friend.

Foreword

We human beings are on the whole extremely trusting of authority. It is, I suspect, something to do with having once been an infant, where trust is the almost inevitable product of having been looked after by people who were sensed as all-powerful and whose care was good enough to ensure our survival. Our total dependence on and reverence for these all-powerful care-givers sets a mould for our later dealings with authority which is broken, often, only with the greatest difficulty and trepidation.

However this may be, and though we may be suspicious and prickly to a degree with almost everyone else, when it comes to those we regard as authorities, our readiness to trust seems almost boundless. In a well-functioning, essentially benign society, this no doubt has its advantages: things run more smoothly if those charged with the direction and care of others (and doing a good job of it) are not questioned mistrustfully at every turn.

However, smooth functioning and benignity are far from *necessary* features of society. There are times – and arguably this is one of them – when societies become infused and corrupted by the pursuit of vested interest, and in this case the more power people have within the society, the easier it will be for them to become corrupted, perfectly possibly without their really noticing it. Those having authority of one kind or another within the society will of course be among those particularly vulnerable to such corruption.

The problem is that, because of our apparently in-built trustfulness, it takes a very long time for the vast majority of us to credit the possibility that the authorities who shape and mediate our culture could in any fundamental sense be mistaken or misleading, let alone corrupt. However conspicuously naked our emperors, we still manage to screw our eyes tight shut and imagine them impeccably decked out in the regalia of their office. Apart, that is, from one or two clear-sighted spectators who, for reasons almost impossible to fathom, are both unable to fool themselves and unable to keep their mouths shut.

Being a vocal witness to nakedness is not a comfortable role to find oneself in. Almost nobody likes a whistle-blower. It attracts neither honour nor thanks. It tends to upset the credulous as much as it infuriates those it exposes. Not only are whistle-blowers likely to be the object of censure and disqualification by the established social institutions which are threatened by their clarity of vision, but they will also find themselves disbelieved and derided by their fellow citizens. The most likely response to a blast from the whistle is a hail of stones from those who, did they but know it, stand to gain most from the truth.

It is easy to anticipate the likely reactions to this book from those whose interests it challenges: it will be labelled as biased, ill-informed, inaccurate, its author as bitter, cynical, off her head. Should it become necessary (i.e., should mere silence not bury the book effectively), there will be no shortage of heavyweight experts lining up to denounce it. For, in testifying to the nakedness of the psychology industry, Tana Dineen finds herself up against a very powerful cultural empire indeed. Never has psychology been more booming and successful. Its wardrobe of imaginary garb is vast and varied, and in the climate of so-called 'post-modernity' it is absolutely central to maintaining a culture of make-believe which distracts us from the harsh realities of our times (harsh, that is, for all but a small minority). This is a nude of Gargantuan proportions.

Rather as Ivan Illich did when, in medicine, he took on an even mightier power,[1] Tana Dineen clearly realized that no mere polemic was going to be enough. This book is tightly argued and meticulously researched. It is difficult to dismiss. But having lived with its North American version for the past three years, Tana Dineen will be only too aware that her efforts are unlikely to be greeted with unstinted approbation and gratitude. And one of the simplest ways to attempt to negate its relevance to a British readership would be to suggest that things over here are not the same as in North America. This, however, is not the case.

As far, at least, as the English-speaking world is concerned, psychology is international, its methods and its preoccupations widely accepted and adopted within the relevant scientific and professional community. The historical background Tana Dineen sketches so skilfully and succinctly in Chapter Six applies as much to Britain as it does to the United States, and the professional activities and aspirations of clinicians, therapists and counsellors across the Atlantic will be instantly recognizable to their British counterparts (as indeed they will to members of the lay public who take an interest in these areas). The only difference, of course, is that, as in pretty well every other area of cultural life, America sets the pace for the anglophone world, leaving the rest of us lagging by a variable period: sometimes years, but sometimes by not much longer than it takes to send an e-mail.

Psychologists and psychotherapists, particularly of course those working within the broadly clinical field, have not in Britain got as far down the line of independent, private practice as they have in the United States, and so far have no statutory form of registration or licensing. But not for want of trying. The British Psychological Society has for some time been pressing government to set up a system of regulation for psychologists somewhat along the lines of that operated in medicine, and various interest groups within the psychotherapy market have, also for years, been struggling to set up regulatory bodies of one kind or another.

So far, the only registers and charters in existence, set up by the professions themselves, are all of a voluntary nature, and employers, for example in the National Health Service, do not require employees to be registered in any way. The pressure is mounting, particularly from the professionals themselves, but also from the media, to introduce statutory regulation of some kind – all, of course, in the name of protection of patients and clients. However, the story told in this book should give us pause for thought. Regulation, licensing, professionalization: all these 'protections' for the public make, in fact, wonderful Trojan horses for public exploitation.

A further indication that British clinical psychology is firmly set on a route taken by its American counterpart is in the relatively recent introduction of a 'doctorate in clinical psychology' as the qualification to be obtained at the end of training on many postgraduate clinical courses. These courses, which have over the years become based far more on 'technique' than on knowledge, are blatantly aimed more at credibility than at scholarly achievement. This is no doubt inevitable in a market-dominated world. Clinical psychology leads the way in the adulteration of academic standards; a 'doctorate in marketing' cannot be far behind.

The days have long gone when the British could laugh at America for its self-indulgent preoccupation with therapy and counselling. Despite being unable to produce a shred of convincing evidence for the efficacy of their procedures, therapy and counselling have not only become a booming market, but therapists and counsellors are now firmly established in British culture, ready to point for justification of their activities to precisely those observations and arguments criticized so effectively in these pages. 'Counselling' as an appropriate and effective response to public disaster and personal tragedy not only enjoys largely unquestioning acceptance, but has come to be seen as a necessary right of those so afflicted.

Although in Britain we may not yet have witnessed some of the psychological excesses described in this book, Tana Dineen's is far more than a cautionary tale. It is above all an unflinching critique of an entire 'scientific' discipline and an exposé of the way it has become corrupted by the vested interests of its practitioners. For psychology did once struggle to be scientific, which, among other things, means to respect evidence. (This is why the professionalization of psychology and the registration of therapists, etc., is so dishonest

– there is no *evidence* that these 'professional' procedures have any real substance.) This book is all about evidence.

It is also about the ethical stance once taken seriously within psychology. This, even though perhaps naively, was to use psychological insights in the interests of the general populace, not merely of psychologists themselves. This book very clearly defends that stance.

Tana Dineen is, then, no mere 'anti-psychologist' – she is psychology's champion. Her work is living proof that psychology is, at least, not quite dead yet. With great good fortune, there may still be enough psychologists around whose respect for evidence and ethical concern will rescue psychology from the dangerously destructive path it has set itself upon. They will take heart from this book.

David Smail
March 1999

Introduction

> *Of all the tyrannies a tyranny sincerely exercised for the good of its victims may be the most oppressive . . . To be cured against one's will and of states which we may not regard as disease is to be put on the level with those who have not yet reached the age of reason or those who never will; to be classed with infants, imbeciles and domestic animals.*
>
> C. S. Lewis

Psychology presents itself as a concerned and caring profession working for the good of its clients. But in its wake lie damaged people, divided families, distorted justice, destroyed companies and a weakened society. Behind the benevolent façade is a voracious, self-serving industry that proffers 'facts' which are often unfounded, provides 'therapy' which can be damaging, and exerts influence which is having devastating effects on the social fabric. The foundation of modern psychology, its critical thinking, if not an illusion from its inception, has now been largely abandoned in favour of power and profit, leaving only the guise of integrity, a show of arrogance and a well-tuned attention to the bottom line. What seemed once a responsible profession is now a big business whose success is directly related to how many people become 'users'.

I was first drawn to the study of psychology by a fascination with human nature, the complexity of life, the content of consciousness and the richness of symbols. Being both curious and sceptical, I was inclined to ask questions, to look for alternative explanations and to challenge assumptions. While I have enjoyed the research and the clinical work of the past thirty years, I have noted, with increasing distress, a shift within psychology from questions to answers, from curiosity to certainty, from modesty to pretentiousness. I now distance myself from my profession, preferring to use the pronoun 'they' when referring to psychologists. For me, there can be no pride associated with belonging to a group which is intent on interfering in people's lives as it promotes its own interests under the guise of an established science and the deceptive image of a responsible profession.

Among my early teachers were the psychologist Donald Hebb and the neurosurgeon Wilder Penfield. Both taught, by example, the excitement of exploring human mysteries and the importance of maintaining a clear distinction between knowledge and speculation. I can still remember Hebb talking to me about the science of psychology, both its possibilities and its limitations. He was fond of stating that psychology was 'more than common sense' and of explaining that he was not implying that psychologists have access to any fund of superior knowledge but rather insisting on an obligation to weigh and examine all issues in a cautious, scientific manner and to remember always that current knowledge is imperfect.

It was in 1969, while developing a system to monitor and evaluate psychiatric services in a general hospital, that I had my first glimpse of professionals acting as if they had access to some hidden fund of superior knowledge. The extreme confidence of many of the psychiatrists disturbed me. It seemed that there was no room in their minds for doubts and no space for questions. I became wary of their judgements and concerned about the impact of their opinions on people's lives. My research over the next few years looked into how psychiatrists went about deciding what was wrong with their patients and what treatment was needed. When I began systematically to examine their decision-making, it became evident that personal beliefs and subjective theories, especially about the causes of problems, influenced their diagnoses and treatments more than did any available information about individual patients, including observable symptoms and verifiable histories.[1] My findings became part of a growing body of scientific literature which at that time was being used to challenge the patriarchal authority of the psychiatric profession.

Later, as I moved into clinical work, I tried to ignore the continual flow of beliefs disguised as findings, the psychological fads promoted as the latest discoveries and the spread of 'pop psychology'. Over the years, I met some very disturbed people who needed help and even protection. However, most of the patients who came to my office in recent years I would refuse to categorize in this way. I would consider it dishonest to declare them 'sick', harmful to label them traumatized or damaged, and disrespectful to treat them as less competent, capable or mature than people I meet in other contexts.

Unfortunately the influence of the Psychology Industry now extends across all aspects of life, telling us how to work, how to live, how to love and even how to play. We are confronted by psychologists expounding their theories on the endless list of TV talk shows, in broadcast news and in the supermarket tabloids, on subjects as wide-ranging as the 'recaps' of celebrity trials or the epidemics of post-traumatic stress disorders after disasters.

Meanwhile, people who are mildly anxious, slightly unhappy or just plain bored are turning more and more to psychology for relief. Some do this through weekly appointments; others by frequenting seminars and workshops; others by endlessly buying books on 'abuse', 'trauma', 'stress' and 'recovery'; all in the pursuit of an elusive experience held out, like a carrot or a pot of gold, by the Psychology Industry.

It is not news to say that psychology has become an influential force or that society is becoming more and more filled with people who consider themselves victims of one sort or another.

What *is* news is that psychology is manufacturing most of these victims; that it is doing this with motives based on power and profit.

The recovered memory/false memory controversy, which has raged over recent years, has served as a major stimulus of scepticism in the courts and in the general public regarding psychology. The shock reverberating through the 'industry' as more and more accusations are being identified as false and prominent court decisions are being overturned, suggests that soon, for the first time in history, a psychological product will actually be declared harmful and withdrawn from the therapeutic shelf. 'Recovered memory therapy' (RMT) is undeniably under attack as serious damages to individuals, families and the court system are being recognized.[2]

However, the public needs to recognize that what has been exposed is just the tip of the iceberg. While important in and of itself, remaining focused on RMT must not distract attention away from the fact that it is just one example of a much larger, generalized business of manufacturing victims. While people have become used to hearing about all sorts of victims, from those of sexual harassment and verbal abuse, to those of 'dysfunctional families', divorce, academic discrimination, even vacation cancellation and home renovation, they have not yet paid attention to the psychological techniques which are being used to create and cater to these 'victims'. Nor have they noticed how it is the psychologists who are benefiting in the end from this victim-making, as the industry creates 'users' dependent on their services.

Whether psychologists ply their trade in a direct manner by assessing and treating people's problems or in an indirect fashion as experts in courts, consultants to government or spokespersons to the media, they foster and promote the positive public image of themselves as caring and powerful. What the Psychology Industry wants people to believe is that it 'knows what is best' and that it has special skills which enable it to 'know what is true'. For example, the psychiatrist Judith Herman wrote in the popular book *Trauma and Recovery*:

> The therapist becomes the patient's ally, placing all the resources of her knowledge, skill, and experience at the patient's disposal . . . The patient enters therapy in *need of help and care*. By virtue of this fact, she voluntarily submits herself to an unequal relationship in which the therapist has *superior status and power*.[3]

But the Psychology Industry is not an ally at all; it is a self-serving business determined to extend its influence, expand its markets and increase its overall profits. It intends that people accept their need for psychology, assume an inferior and dependent role, and become 'users'. It is through caring that psychologists create need, and through helping that they establish dependency.

Consider the following apparently disparate cases:

- A toll-free number, promoted nationally, offers psychological help if people consider themselves 'victims of the Oklahoma City Bombing', while locally, psychologists develop a public-education campaign 'to turn this disaster into something productive for survivors so they don't feel their loved ones died in vain'.[4]
- A team of social workers which travelled to the Middle East to identify and treat the psychological casualties of Operation Desert Storm report on the benefits of their work, concluding that 'early recognition of the traumatic experiences will assist veterans in seeking treatment sooner and developing an awareness of stress in themselves and family members.'[5]
- The American Psychological Association using 'rape as a barometer of female fear', stating that there is 'no safe haven' for women, recommends collecting more data on female-directed violence and advocates the development of 'more innovative treatment' for both female victims and male perpetrators.[6]
- The Canadian Register of Health Service Providers in Psychology reports on the success of 'a cardiovascular marketing project' designed to promote psychology as 'an authoritative resource, with knowledge, skills and techniques . . . integral to the process of CV illness prevention'.[7]
- A doctor in Vermont states that caffeine is 'a drug of abuse', pointing out that 6 million Americans are unable to quit, and suggesting that 'the mental health community needs the ability to diagnose caffeine abuse and begin developing treatment services.'[8]

- Social workers in California refer to predictions that by the year 2000 the depressed elderly will constitute 13 per cent of the US population and suggest ways social work can take an active role in targeting 'the large pool of elderly clients' in need of treatment.[9]
- A former comedienne completes her PhD dissertation on the deleterious effects of fame on the famous and begins her professional life as a Los Angeles psychologist specializing in 'the anguish of fame'.[10]

What do all these situations have in common? Each of these 'noble' efforts evokes the image of the world as a dangerous place strewn with psychological casualties, and promotes the seemingly humanitarian idea that more psychological services are needed to reduce 'the risks' and tend to 'the wounded'. In all cases, a psychological formula is being applied defining various groups of people as victims who are in need of psychological help. This is the process involved in the manufacturing of victims by the Psychology Industry as it applies its business formula:

PERSON = VICTIM = USER/PATIENT = PROFIT

'Victim', once a term reserved for those who suffered from a calamity of nature, of fate or of violent crime, has become psychologized so that it can be applied broadly to anyone and everyone who knowingly or unknowingly has been exposed to or experienced stress, distress or trauma. Feelings of unhappiness, boredom, anger, sadness and guilt can now all be interpreted as signs of prior trauma, creating victims. Whether these people then pursue treatment, sue their perpetrator or seek expert advice, they all become users of the Psychology Industry, providing its income and increasing its overall asset worth.

Evidence of the current success and growth of the industry can be seen in the number of Americans becoming users. In the early 1960s, 14 per cent of the US population (25 million) had received some psychological service. By 1976, that number had risen to 26 per cent;[11] by 1990, to 33 per cent. And by 1995, according to the American Psychological Association, 46 per cent (128 million) had seen a mental-health professional. Some predict that by early in the twenty-first century, users will be the majority – constituting 80 per cent of the population.[12]

There are many incentives for acquiring, and even for seeking, victim status and, in the short term, there are pay-offs. The tragedies, the failures, the hardships, the health problems and the disappointments of life become explained, relieving people of at least three of life's natural burdens: dealing with complexity, facing things beyond their control, and accepting personal responsibility for decisions and actions. The newest psychological technologies promise relief from these and also give people who have led the dullest of lives a thread of meaning or a dash of excitement. Lives that seem shamefully ordinary take on a melodramatic quality. Victim stories flow into conversations, becoming the excuses for the embarrassments, regrets or failures of people's lives. For some, including many of the most prominent in the industry, victim status itself is the credential which qualifies them as psychologists.[13] For these entrepreneurs and for many others, being a victim opens the door to a successful career.

Near the beginning of the twentieth century it was suggested that 'Psychologists should . . . take the place of doctors, counsellors, fortune tellers, and relatives',[14] and now, at the dawn of the twenty-first century, it seems that the Psychology Industry has discovered how to achieve this goal. It is because the current business formula is working so well that there is such an urgency now to expose psychology as the irresponsible and out-of-control industry it has become.

What is referred to in this book as the 'Psychology Industry' is still thought by the public to be something quite different from other industries, somehow more noble, honest, and less profit-driven. When people think of industries, they tend to think of automobiles, computers, cosmetics or entertainment; of easily identifiable products, with price tags, guarantees and trademarks. Such industries are visibly defined by their products and by their boundaries. The Psychology Industry is much harder to pin down; it is much broader than other industries, less defined (or definable). At its core, along with the traditional mental-health professions of psychology, psychiatry, psychoanalysis and clinical social work, is a fifth psychological profession: psychotherapy.[15] No longer can clear distinctions be made between them; so, what I call the Psychology Industry comprises all five of these. It also encompasses the ever-expanding array of psychotherapists: the counsellors and advisers of all persuasions. As the American Psychological Association notes: 'The general public often has difficulty in understanding the differences between professional psychologists and *other types of psychologists*, between professional psychologists and psychiatrists, between psychologists and counsellors, or between psychologists and *a variety of other professionals who deal with emotional, health, and behavioral problems*.'[16]

This term acknowledges that around the edges of the industry are other individuals whose work, whether it involves writing, consulting, lecturing or even filmmaking, relies on the Psychology Industry, which in turn benefits from their promotion of all things psychological.

Psychology is not the profession that it claims to be, nor is it just a business like other businesses. It is too big and too dangerous now not to be seen and judged as an industry complete with advertising slogans, sales and marketing programmes, research and development, production and assembly lines, and unions. This is the era of licensed, accredited, certified, proclaimed or self-proclaimed psychologists. With degrees in psychology, medicine, social work, nursing or with no academic qualifications at all, the expanding workforce of the Psychology Industry relies for its survival and growth on its ability to manufacture victims. Specializing in trauma, stress, abuse and addiction, an increasing number of psychologists are competing for 'victim fees'. Few of them ask any questions or show any reservations about their business. Most equate expert status with their own adamant beliefs which, with no pause for critical thought or responsible reflection, they present as 'findings' and 'facts'.

When the term 'psychologist' (with a small 'p') is used in this book, as it is over and over again, it is with reference to this larger and somewhat diffuse group of people. The choice to use the term in this way has annoyed professional organizations, licensing boards and many of my colleagues who wish to protect this title for licensed psychologists. Use of the term has, since the 1950s, become restricted throughout North America and parts of the Commonwealth, with only those having met the requirements of a licensing board being authorized to call themselves psychologists. The argument initially made was that the public would be protected from improperly trained charlatans who, unrestrained by a code of professional ethics, were not trustworthy. The British Psychological Society has long been seeking the statutory restriction of the term 'psychologist' in this way. So far this has resulted only in a voluntary 'charter'. There is little reason to suppose that success in achieving fully restrictive legislation would result in anything very different from the North American experience. As this book shows, the protection of the term has nothing to do with protection of the public. From the beginning it has been used in a self-serving way to bolster a false image, support a business strategy and gain influence. The serious issues of responsible professionalism remain unaddressed.

Having said this, I want to acknowledge that there are some among my colleagues who are not 'in the business'. Not all psychologists are allowing themselves to be swept along by seductive theorizing and popular beliefs. However, while continuing to distinguish fact from opinion and resisting becoming victim-makers themselves, most are hesitating to express their dissenting views. Fearful of jeopardizing their own financial security and reputations, afraid of personal attacks, or concluding that there is nothing they can do, they are choosing to remain silent. There are also those who have continued to take research seriously, acknowledging the limits of their knowledge, and showing respect for people. But this is not because they have a PhD or a licence; it is because of who they are. Some are attempting to save what remains of the science and of the ethical practice of psychology, but a change of this magnitude cannot come from the fraternal organizations which have failed to protect the public and continue to promote the industry. In North America, at least, it is too late. Psychology has become too influential, too bureaucratic, too political; it will never voluntarily relinquish its power.

In the autumn of 1993, after spending an afternoon with a colleague reflecting on what was happening in psychology, I asked, half jokingly, whether he thought that psychologists might soon start leaving the profession the way dissenting priests had, some time ago, begun to leave the church. He thought for a moment and then replied: 'Not a chance. There's too much money in it.'[17] There was not a hint of humour in his voice; his tone was so serious and his manner so sombre that his words stuck in my head.

Psychology has become big business. This business, which presents itself authoritatively in a language that appears to be scientific, has succeeded in turning American society into what Charles Sykes recently termed 'a nation of victims'.[18] In this regard, another term, 'user', is employed throughout this book to identify the broad scope of individuals who either directly or indirectly use the services of the Psychology Industry. It refers not only to those who are clients and patients of psychologists, for some are users even though they may never have visited a psychologist, by virtue of adopting and applying psychologized concepts about behaviours, thoughts and feelings. The examples are so plentiful, so pervasive and so much a part of everyday life that they go unrecognized as the products, the end results of the Psychology Industry.

The American Psychological Association is the largest professional organization representing psychology in the United States. With a 1999 membership of over 155,000, it is also the largest association of psychologists in the world. Since it is such an influential force within the Psychology Industry, frequent reference will be made to it throughout this book; so, for convenience, it will be referred to as the APA.

People smile knowingly at cartoons that appear in daily newspapers and magazines. But they miss the point. Taking on a victim role is no laughing matter. The following examples demonstrate the variety of victims manufactured, serviced and harmed by the industry.

A patient I was seeing for the first time in my clinical practice asked to be hypnotized so that he could discover whatever it was in his past that was making him the way he was now. He had recently watched a television show about satanic ritual abuse which suggested to him that he might be a 'victim' and that finding a buried trauma was '*the* answer'. The man, who had a long psychiatric history, reported that on the way to his appointment with me he had resisted the voices in his head telling him to kill the person standing next to him at the bus stop. He described how he 'enjoyed' sticking sharp objects up his rectum and showed me samples of the bizarre thoughts he had been writing down. His symptoms indicated a biologically based mental illness, schizophrenia. Hypnotizing him seemed both unsafe and inappropriate. But he refused consent for me to see his treatment history, and insisted on an immediate referral to a local licensed psychologist who specialized in 'ritual abuse'. I called her and after a discussion of the case lasting less than a minute, she stated that the man was a victim of satanic ritual abuse and that she could arrange for him to be 'treated'. She had arrived at her instant diagnosis without asking a single question. The patient was – reluctantly – given the referral he had requested. Very early one morning a year later, he called me from a phone booth having been in a hospital emergency department all night receiving thirty stitches, after obeying the voices in his head which had told him to gash himself open with a piece of sharp glass. His psychologist, whom he had been seeing weekly for the year, had recently informed him that his failure to improve was because he required two weekly sessions rather than one to deal with the effects of his ritual abuse. He admitted that he still couldn't remember having been abused in the ways she described. He couldn't afford two sessions a week.

This is but one of many examples in my experience in which psychologists have been bent on applying their formula for profit. The individual becomes 'the victim' and thus 'the patient' who needs ongoing psychological treatment and, in an enterprising rather than scientific way, the failure to achieve success is explained as indicating the need for more, not less.

Examples like this are not found only in clinical practice. For instance, a hairdresser whose warmth had always impressed me suddenly changed; there was no sparkle and no animated conversation. When asked why, she told of discovering that she was a 'victim of incest' and described how memories had begun coming back of how her father had sexually abused her from the time she was six months old. She was in therapy now and that was all she had to talk about. She had lost her vitality and independence, relying on her psychologist to interpret her past, explain her present and predict her future. For the psychologist, a profitable business relationship had been established.

The entrepreneurship can sometimes be quite apparent. For instance, a couple went to a marriage counsellor. At the end of the husband's second session, the psychologist informed him that their marital problems were due to the 'fact' that he was a 'victim of a dysfunctional family'. He had mentioned that his father had often been away from home for work reasons when he was a child and she concluded from this that his father was an alcoholic, which was news to him, and that he should view himself as an 'adult child of an alcoholic' needing long-term treatment. His wife had laughed at him when he told her about his session, refusing to believe that the psychologist could have come to this bizarre conclusion. However, when she next saw the psychologist, she was given the same explanation for their problems. Both she and her husband concluded that the psychologist was dangerous and managed to get away before becoming entangled in her beliefs and trapped in her business.

A young woman told me recently that she was avoiding phone calls from a friend who talked incessantly about her 'wounded inner child'. The descriptions of her friend's stories were reminiscent of a workshop I had attended which was conducted by John Bradshaw, an ex-priest and recovered alcoholic, whose books and national television shows have reached millions of North Americans, telling them about the benefits of getting in touch with their 'inner child'. I had been horrified by the cult-like atmosphere and by the required 'exercises' which basically dictated to people the scripts of their own childhood. In one of these exercises the participants were told to visualize a playground scene and then to rescue their child self. They were informed that if the child resisted, they should drag him or her away from the dark past anyway, kicking and screaming if necessary, into the modern daylight of a therapist's office. An evangelical force had pervaded the room and the standing ovation at the end from the audience of over a thousand, caused me to wonder how many workshops this woman's friend would pay to attend, how many tapes, books and teddy bears she would buy and whether, in the end, she would have any friends left who would not be avoiding her phone calls.

These examples illustrate how victim-making works. Once individuals accept a 'victim' label, their lives become centred on this new identity. Like the hairdresser described earlier, being a victim becomes all they have to think, talk or read about. And it becomes a focus of their spending. They, their friends and society come to believe that everyone needs help whether they know it or not. Instead of a light at the end of the tunnel, now there is a psychologist waiting to be paid.

Some time ago, a seventeen-year-old girl in a small town was hit by a car and killed. The parents were overwhelmed with sadness. One of their neighbours suggested that the community take up a collection to pay for grief counselling for the parents. Instantly the surviving parents, rather than the dead girl, had become identified as 'the victims'. And just as quickly, they were being cast into a 'patient' role, becoming part of the market for all the books, articles and courses about the 'normal' stages of grieving which package raw human emotions into sanitized psychological stages. Would it not be better to consider what had happened as a tragic event and what these parents were going through as their own private, and quite inconsolable, feelings of sadness and loss? Would it not be better to let them turn to God or to each other? But grieving and mourning are no longer within the domain of either family or religion. The Psychology Industry has corralled them, marketing them as a psychological process to be carried out under expert supervision. Now anyone who is suffering is viewed as a victim. Society has accepted the bizarre idea that there must be some psychological solution to all of life's pain and that for a price one can buy it for oneself or even purchase it as a gift.

Some psychologists have focused recently on war veterans as victims of unresolved traumas, describing how, half a century after the end of the Second World War, the ageing veterans were having traumatic memories triggered by anniversary celebrations. One article gives as an example a 72-year-old veteran, recently diagnosed as suffering from 'post-traumatic stress disorder'. After describing his nightmares and the guilt he was feeling over having killed a young German soldier by slashing his throat with a bayonet, the writer comments: 'Now a half century later only one of them can rest in peace . . .' But why call the surviving war veteran a victim? Why turn his moral turmoil into a psychological illness? Could it be that the Psychology Industry sees a potential market here to create some new demand for services? Could it be that the toll-free number at the end of this article, which invited 'veterans experiencing sleeplessness, anxiety, crying spells, flashbacks, depression or heavy drinking' to call for help, is part of a marketing scheme?[19] It may sound cynical, but remember that the Psychology Industry needs 'users'.

Much as the marketing of Rolex watches or Gucci bags has led to the emergence of frauds and counterfeits, the psychological mass marketing of the victim has produced its own counterfeits. For example, a bank teller described the problems she was having with her daughter. The girl, who was seeing a social worker because she was flagrantly disobeying the rules at home and at school, had threatened to make up a story about how her new stepfather was sexually abusing her. Unless her mother agreed to let her stay out as late as she liked, buy anything she wanted and do anything she pleased, she would tell her social worker the story. The newly remarried mother was horrified and her new husband was terrified. They had both read too many newspaper reports about people being criminally charged on the basis of such stories and they were trying to find a way to deal with being held hostage under this threat of 'crying victim'.

The word 'victim' used to evoke images of blood and torn limbs on a battlefield, naked bodies thrown into a mass grave, scenes of torture, terrible accidents, brutal murders and violent rapes. These harsh images, which defined the word, have now been fused with fuzzy images of people grieving, expressing regrets, hugging teddy bears or demanding retribution. Certainly there are people today who can be recognized in terms of the harsh, rather than the fuzzy, images. One who comes quickly to my mind is a little boy in Truillo, Peru. He walked up to me one sunny day as I was sitting on a bench in the town square. He glanced with curiosity at my Spanish dictionary and pointed to my shoes, offering to shine them for what would have amounted to a few pennies. Wanting to learn something about his life, I asked him, in Spanish, to sit for a minute and talk with me. He told me that he was eight years old, had no idea who his parents were, and lived on the streets; he couldn't write his name and he had no address. He pointed to a man watching us from across the square, saying that he was the boss to whom he and the other kids like him reported. He explained that by shining enough shoes during the day he could earn something to eat at night. He said that often he didn't earn enough, sometimes going days with nothing to eat. He showed me the scars and fresh burn marks on his hands and arms, saying that he'd have more of these if he didn't get back to work. He smiled and waved goodbye as he ran off across the square seeking another customer. That was his life; every day he struggled to survive. But that little boy was alert to what was going on around him and he was very much alive.

I think of him often, and sometimes I wonder what happened to him and whether, by some miracle, he managed to escape. In many years of clinical practice, I have seen a number of patients who are authentic survivors, many of accidents, some of crimes, and a few of situations a bit similar to his.

Some time ago, a young woman came to my office with a specific request. She was a Christian Iranian, who had grown up in Teheran, where she had married and had a child, a daughter. Her husband, university educated, had worked for a small newspaper. One day, the Iranian police had come to her parents' home, where the young couple lived, and arrested them as traitors. She was taken to a prison where she remained for eight months, repeatedly being interrogated about her husband's activities. While in prison, she heard of her husband's torture and execution. Eventually she was released and, with her parents' help, escaped with her daughter, arriving in Canada as a political refugee. She held little hope that she would ever again see her family, her friends, or anything of the life that had been familiar to her. Despite the vivid experiences she described of brutality, torture, cruelty and murder, and in spite of the fear, nightmares, loneliness and loss that she experienced, she spoke with a thread of life running through her words. This, all of it, was her life. Now she had learned a new language, succeeded in being accepted into university, and wanted help to develop ways to control feelings of panic that occasionally intruded, interfering with her concentration. She made it clear that she wanted to create a new life for herself, far different from what she had imagined, but still a life. She was a 'survivor' already, so why call her a victim? To insist that she needed to explore her past trauma and deal with it in some psychologically endorsed manner would be to ignore her own resilience and to undermine what she had accomplished already on her own. Responding to her request meant expressing respect and admiration for how well she had done and suggesting some simple ways to put the feelings of panic aside whenever they began to interfere with her studying. The last time we met she talked about how well she was doing in her course work and what plans she had for the next school year. One can only hope that over the years, during some moment of uncertainty, she will not become the prey of a psychologist who, with the arrogance which has come to replace judgement, makes her a victim by convincing her to go back.

Given the determination she displayed from the first, it seems likely that she would have the strength to resist such a sales pitch. It is possible that, although everyone has moments of weakness, those who have survived such experiences as hers are actually better able than most to resist psychological influence. While occasionally they make big news, authentic victims are not big business. They tend not to be good raw material for the type of victim-making profitable to psychologists.

In the Psychology Industry, it is generally recognized that there is not much money to be made, nor glory to be gained, by working with readily identifiable victims. And the poor, the homeless and those working and struggling either to survive, like the Peruvian boy, or to go on with life, like the Iranian woman, are unlikely to have the money or the time to indulge in 'recovery'. So, as far as the Psychology Industry goes, unless there is some funding source to tap, most authentic victims and survivors go unnoticed.

It is the fabricated victims rather than the real ones who are big news and big business. Granted, stories of authentic victims tend to preface the scripts of those being cultivated as 'users', causing the various new forms of 'victims' to seem just the same. But the word 'victim' has a new, diluted meaning. Drawing its thrust from association with actual atrocities such as the Holocaust, the word is now closely connected to the popular psychologized versions of 'emotional trauma'. 'Victim', as used by psychologists, frequently refers to someone who is momentarily upset or generally less satisfied, less happy, less successful or less fulfilled than they believe they should be and who attributes that feeling to something supposedly done to them, or merely witnessed or worried about.

Virtually any event can now qualify a person as a victim. There are the dramatic varieties such as the alleged victims of satanic ritual abuse or of UFO abductions. Then there are the more everyday varieties such as victims of shopping addiction and verbal abuse. To be declared a victim of sexual assault can now mean anything from having been abducted and repeatedly raped at knifepoint to having had an affair with a professor which ended with a grade that wasn't the expected A, having got drunk one night and gone to bed with a date who looked less appealing in the sober morning light, or even having been whistled at. To be declared a victim of violence can mean anything from having been dragged into a dark lane and beaten to death, to having been slapped during a quarrel or becoming upset after hearing news of a subway accident or watching a violent scene in a movie. Psychologists say that whatever happened, 'the experience', which they translate into psychological effects, can be equally devastating.

The following quote provides an illustration:

> Every victim of personal crime is confronted with a brutal reality: the deliberate violation of one human being by another. The crime may be a murder or a rape, a robbery or a burglary, the theft of an automobile, a pocket picking or a purse snatching – but *the essential internal injury is the same.* Victims have been assaulted emotionally and sometimes physically by a predator who *has shaken their world to its foundations.*[20]

Stereotyping of this magnitude is offensive not only because it overlooks human strength, courage and resilience, ignores those who might be capable of dealing with the theft of a wallet, and insults the authentic victims who have endured what most of us cannot even imagine, but also because it misuses science, misleads the public and eludes basic common sense. That such statements, when made by psychologists, are taken seriously and that such ideas now pervade our culture, demonstrates the power of psychological marketing.

A popular bumper sticker used to read 'Trust me, I'm a doctor.' Recently the psychological equivalent was expressed on a national news programme but this time with all seriousness: 'He has to know; after all he is a psychologist!' The medical version long ago became a joke. But the radio announcer wasn't laughing when she referred to the psychologist in this same naive way. She seemed actually to believe that anyone who calls themselves a psychologist has insight, special knowledge and understanding, and an unswerving allegiance to truth. The image she held in her mind was the prevailing one of psychology as 'a caring profession'.

Manufacturing Victims challenges that image. It presents psychology as an industry – the business of turning people into victims. In recent years, I have come to accept an ethical obligation not only to dissociate myself from this business but also to take whatever action I can to curb its influence. I find it no longer possible to ignore the spewing of psychological 'facts', 'interpretations' and 'solutions' and to avoid facing the vast scope of their pernicious influence. In some ways, this book is my apology for decades of biting my lip. It takes a cold, hard look at the damaging effects that psychologists are having on individuals and on society.

This book intends to expose psychology as an industry out to sell services, gain influence and make money at the expense of both the authentic victims, which it fails to respect or to protect, and of the fabricated victims manufactured by it. The Psychology Industry is a North-American invention whose influence has spread rapidly across the United States and Canada. Thus, most examples are drawn from this region of the world. However, it should be noted that, like many industries which trace their origin to the United States, the Psychology Industry has been spreading its influence beyond North America. To date, its damaging effects are being felt primarily in western Europe, especially in Britain and the Netherlands, and in Australia and New Zealand.

Chapter One outlines the psychological techniques employed in victim-making, illustrating how these techniques have led to a wide acceptance of erroneous beliefs about 'the typical victim'. It concludes with a description of the stereotypical victim image which serves as a mould for fabricating victims. Chapter Two looks at three types of fabricated victims: 1) *synthetic victims*, who are being cast in a variety of victim roles by procedures which influence their memories of the past, experiences of the present and expectations of the future; 2) *contrived victims*, who become caught up in popularized ideas about the psychological causes and consequences of medical conditions such as cancer and heart disease; and 3) *counterfeit victims*, who turn to psychology for validation of their self-determined victim states.

The remainder of the book is about the industry which manufactures them. Chapter Three challenges the public image of psychology as a science, illustrating the industry's misuse and abuse of science and its tendency to ignore studies which undermine its claims and suggest negative effects on individuals and on society. Chapter Four examines how the Psychology Industry accomplishes its business goals by turning life into a series of psychological problems necessitating treatment, impressing society with a plethora of specialities and credentials, and making its services both accessible and essential. Chapter Five discusses a trend towards psychological mechanization, identifying the industrial and often unskilled aspects of the industry, from the simplistic generalizations found in such processes as 'healthy grieving' and 'recovery' through the 'one-concept-fits-all' approach of abuse and addiction counselling, to the franchising and supervising activities of some psychologists. Chapter Six looks at the history of the industry, describing how it became an integral part of the industrial free-enterprise society and how, amid the economic recession and depressive mood of the 1980s, it shifted its efforts into the manufacture of victims.

Chapter Seven takes a final look at the long shadow which the Psychology Industry has cast over human life and human relationships. Offering no simple solutions, it does suggest some ways in which individuals and governments can resist this ominous threat.

Given the strong economic and political roots of this industry and the extent to which the public has become enamoured of what it sells, I harbour no delusions that this book will bring down the industry. I am fully aware that many psychologists and a large number of those people who have learned to see themselves and the world through a psychological lens will not look with favour upon it. Thus, I am prepared for the book to be ignored, dismissed and even condemned.

However, I hope that it will encourage others to begin looking at the practice of psychology differently. And to reassert their right to think for themselves and persist in their questioning of the statements that psychologists make, demanding research in place of rhetoric and logic in place of persuasion. The book offers meat for arguments. I would like to see sensible people challenge the authority, power and privilege of the purported psychological experts of this era, curb the damages being done by psychologists, diminish the influence of the Psychology Industry, and succeed in taking back their own lives.

1
Victim-Making

The therapists transformed age-old human dilemmas into psychological problems and claimed that they (and they alone) had the treatment . . . The result was an explosion of inadequacy.

Charles Sykes

Often I have the feeling of being on the other side of the looking-glass; like Alice, I am trying to make sense of distortions, exaggerations and deceptions. We live in a world of illusion, where our grasp on reality is often tenuous. Artificial wedding cakes look real; actors posing as doctors prescribe cough remedies; old movies are colourized; special effects appear believable; and the world of 'virtual reality' becomes our new reality. Victim-making is part of this world of fabrications and illusions.

With today's distortion of the term 'victim' and the endless proliferation of pretenders, it may seem impossible to distinguish real victims from fabricated varieties. But if one makes an effort to flee the psychological domain with all its misleading statements, misinformation and outright lies about what it means to be a victim, it is possible to know the difference.

From ancient times to today's newspaper, fate and cruelty have affected humanity. Reports of the earthquake in Kobe, Japan, the bombing in Oklahoma City, the shootings in Dunblane, the genocide in Rwanda or the atrocities committed by Jeffery Dahmer, Fred and

Rosemary West or Paul Bernardo, are reminders of a cruel and terrifying side of nature and of human nature which cannot be controlled or eliminated. They are incontrovertible evidence of our vulnerability and they cause naive notions of limitless security to crumble. The experiences of real victims, as well as creating discomfort, bring into question the psychological practice of victim-making; they bring us back from a psychological 'virtual reality' to the tangible reality in which we live out our lives.

The situations in which people become victims span the whole gamut from local tragedies to global genocides. Consider the following three stories; one of a rape victim, the second of a holocaust survivor, and the third of a man whose life was shattered by a car accident.

In July 1992 the Canadian news media reported the mysterious disappearance of a young woman. Screams led police to the place where she was found, tied and bound. For nine days she had been held captive, the victim of a rapist and killer.

It had all begun when, at the end of her shift, right outside the store where she worked, she was abducted at gunpoint. A man forced her to go to a makeshift camp in a wooded area where he tied her ankles, bound her hands behind her back, and shoved a piece of torn blanket into her mouth. When she slept, she did so tied up in a cramped position on the hard ground; when he left her alone she was hog-tied in such a way that her muscles were painfully stretched. He fed her sporadically and occasionally took her for short walks. He held her there, unable to move and naked for most of the time, forcing her to perform whatever sexual acts he demanded. As she later described it:

> The most common and most painful position was with me on my hands and knees, my face pushed right into the ground and him raping me from behind. This resulted in unbelievable pain in my lower back. The best way I can explain it is to imagine someone taking two bones in your back and rubbing them together with extreme pressure . . . My jaw was also very sore for about a month

> from a combination of him hitting me in the face and forcing me to perform oral sex on him.[1]

In her 'victim impact statement' she referred to the discomfort and pain at the time and described bruises and injuries which eventually healed and aches which persisted. She spoke of the pain of simple movements like tying her shoes, sitting down and picking things off the floor as being continuing reminders of what she had endured. She spoke, as well, of her inability to 'put into words how terrifying it feels to have someone take control of your life'.

The second story is of the Holocaust survivor and Nobel Prize winner Elie Wiesel. He knows well how difficult it is to try to put such experiences into words. His first book, *Night*, is a thin volume which relates his memories from before his arrest at the age of fourteen to his release from Buchenwald at the end of the war. Wiesel describes a reality which 'he saw and touched and tasted directly'.[2] He records how he and his family were marched from the ghetto to the train station, where they were loaded into a cattle cars. When the train arrived at Birkenau, the reception centre for Auschwitz, he watched as his mother and his young sister were forced to walk to the right while he and his father were ordered to walk in the other direction. His mother and sister were burned in the crematory; he and his father watched the flames and the smoke. Three weeks later they were transferred to Buna, where prisoners were ordered to strip naked and run in front of the notorious Dr Mengele so that he could 'examine' them, selecting those whose physical condition was more suited for execution than continued labour. He described his life at that time thus: 'These were terrible days. We received more blows than food; we were crushed with work.'[3]

Months later Wiesel was in an infirmary bed with a severely injured foot when the rumour spread that the camp was to be evacuated. It was assumed that the SS guards would execute all those who were unable to walk; so he got up and marched with the others out the gates of the camp. The wind was icy. It snowed relentlessly. The SS had orders to shoot anyone who could not keep up. Near him men, collapsing in the dirty snow, were being shot. He kept repeating to himself: 'Don't think. Don't stop. Run.'

After a train ride, during which those already dead and those about to die were periodically thrown from the car to reduce the stench, Wiesel and his father arrived at Buchenwald. His father, his only reason throughout the entire ordeal to keep going, had been struck down with dysentery. On 28 January the boy climbed into his bunk above his father and in the morning: 'I awoke on January 29 at dawn. In my father's place lay another invalid. They must have taken him away before dawn and carried him to the crematory. He may still have been breathing.'[4]

The third story is of an accident victim who consulted me on the first anniversary of the event which had shattered his life. What he described was not a part of history; it was not even the kind of story that gets into the newspaper. He was a middle-aged Italian immigrant who had worked hard as a truck driver for twenty years before finally getting a job in a packing plant. In tearful, broken English, he described how he had been alone in his car, driving home, when he saw the lights of a transport truck coming at him. The truck hit him head on, totally demolishing his car, crashing his head into the windshield and smashing his right arm. He was unconscious when he arrived at the emergency room. The arm was not set properly; no one seemed concerned about his head injury. His arm remained visibly deformed and a bone literally stuck out from his wrist. He described the pain, the dizziness and the flashes of light inside his head that kept him awake through the night, and said he was unable to do anything he used to do, such as shovel snow, drive a car, remember an appointment or even follow a conversation. He spoke of how he avoided going to visit friends or even talking with his family because he feared 'looking stupid'. People had kept telling him that he would get better; he was beginning to doubt that he ever would.

This man, the young woman and Elie Wiesel are victims. Each of them has experienced something out of the ordinary; each of them speaks of what happened in the past, putting into words his or her own thoughts, feelings and reactions; those who want to understand what it means to be a victim can learn by listening respectfully to them.

But the Psychology Industry uses and abuses the experiences of people such as these, in order to further its own business interests. In order to thrive, the Psychology Industry requires an ever-expanding number of fabricated victims. The three principles on which the modern day mass production of victims relies are:

Psychologizing – using psychological constructs to reduce real experiences to theories, thus making the external world a figment of an unconscious and subjective inner realm. The Psychology Industry pretends to understand the unconscious and, thus, to be able to accurately interpret what victims experience.

Pathologizing – turning, with psychological arrogance, ordinary (and extraordinary) people in abnormal (seemingly unbearable) situations into 'abnormal' people, labelling all victims 'damaged', 'wounded', 'abused', 'traumatized', incapable of dealing with it, getting over it or going on with life. The Psychology Industry claims the authority to deduce psychological illness and harm, to cut through to uncertainties, vulnerabilities and regrets, and to diagnose, categorize and label human experience.

Generalizing – equating the exceptional and the brutal with the ordinary and the mundane, thus ignoring the differences which set victims apart in an insulting effort to extend and blur them with the more common experiences of a lifetime. The Psychology Industry assumes the capacity to psychologize the mundane, using metaphor to create an absurd realm of similarities, equating the thought with the deed, the dream with the fact, and the illusion with the reality.

Through these techniques, it reduces the complex fabric of life to a single thread, turning the whole gamut of human qualities into psychologically defined 'processes'. All this psychologizing, pathologizing and generalizing is done for the purpose of victim-making, patient-making – user-making.

Psychologizing

Treating the medical metaphors of modern psychiatry as literal reflects and reinforces our modern aversion to moral conflict, human tragedy, and plain language.[5]

Psychologizing turns what individual victims say about events and their effects into ideas which are very different and even disconnected from the victims' descriptions. Presenting these ideas as facts, psychologists can then apply them to other peoples' lives, transforming virtually anyone into a victim. Psychologizing assumes as its basis an interior world in which an unconscious has profound influence, a place where things are different from what they seem on the outside. And it relies on the belief that, like guides familiar with the terrain, psychologists can see what is hidden there: what is not known (about the past), what can't be seen (in the present), and what must be discovered (to achieve a better future).

Psychologizing involves:

1) constructing a theory about victimization,
2) applying that theory to individuals,
3) turning personal events into psychological symbols, which are expressed in psychological language,
4) creating the need for psychologists who can interpret the symbols.

Psychology has created numerous theories in an attempt to explain both the similarities and the differences in people's actions and reactions. In the past, psychological theories were developed by researchers who, through scientific methods, addressed such issues as perception (e.g. the ability to see differences in colours) and behaviour (e.g. the use of rewards or reinforcement to change reactions). Today the theories of the Psychology Industry are more likely to be developed by practitioners on the basis of their experience with patients and to be accepted despite being untested by any scientific means. It is these clinical theories that are presented as the latest, the most up-to-date explanations of the causes of problems and serve to demonstrate the need for 'healing' and 'recovery'.

These theories are applied either directly to individuals through psychological consultations when patients are led to believe that they have experienced trauma, or indirectly by experts who speak of hypothetical cases. For instance, in a high-profile Canadian criminal case, that of Paul Bernardo, charged with the abduction, repeated rape and gruesome murder of two teenage girls, experts applied their theories. Two psychologists testified about 'battered wife syndrome' as it might hypothetically apply to Bernardo's ex-wife's involvement and complicity in the case. The theory was introduced in an effort to cast her as a psychological victim rather than an accomplice. As often happens, the supposed victim of this hypothetical syndrome was never interviewed or even seen by the experts. Rather, the psychologists applied the syndrome as a template in an attempt to explain the behaviour of a woman they had never met.

Through the application of theories, psychologists can turn the specific events, feelings and thoughts of people's lives into psychological symbols and esoteric language. According to Martin Gross, America has become a 'psychological society' in which psychologists are allowed, even expected, to interpret what people say, feel and do, and to explain their words, moods and actions.[6] It has come to be accepted that what happens to people on the 'outside' has an effect on the 'inside' and that it is what happens on the 'inside' that determines their lives. This psychological concept holds remarkable similarity to the astrological idea that what happens in the sky determines what happens in people's lives. Both rely on the assumed ability of trained, gifted or selected people who can see either what is written in the sky or what is hidden in the unconscious. The practitioners of both speak and act as if they are members of a secret society in which they have been taught to see and hear at a deeper level. They translate external events into their own esoteric language and attribute profound influences to them. And in doing so they cause themselves to be held in awe and their services to be in demand.

Just as glossolalia (speaking in tongues) of the early Christian Church created the need for those with the 'gift of interpretation', the esoteric psychological jargon creates the need for psychologists who can explain and cure the problems. Calling it 'expertise', psychologists claim an ability to see the inner worlds of other people. Focusing on what they believe is happening on the inside and minimizing the importance of what is happening on the outside, psychologists say with assumed confidence: '*I know* how you really feel'; '*I know* what you're really saying'; '*I know* how badly you've been hurt', '*I know* what really happened to you.' And the uninitiated consumer, hesitates to ask: 'How do you know?' or to say: 'You're wrong.' So psychologists get away with applying their theories, with their psychologizing and with their victim-making.

Psychologizing

VICTIMS ==> THEORIES

these theories are then used to turn

VICTIMS <== PEOPLE

Consider again the example in the Introduction in which the psychologist instantly, and quite magically, determined that a man had been tortured by satanists. The only information given her was that the man looked anxious, claimed to hear voices, reported having done bizarre things to himself and had watched a television show about ritual abuse. He had no memory of any 'satanic ritual abuse' but *she knew* that he was a victim of it. She described in amazing detail how 'they' had tortured him. Without hesitation and without asking a single question, she claimed to *know* what had happened and declared that he needed help to recover these memories to be cured; help that she could offer. This psychologist demonstrated none of the finely tuned skills of listening on which the popular acceptance of psychologists' power has been based. Instead of asking about his life and making some effort to understand what was happening to this particular man, she presumed a psychologized theory of ritual abuse. Never having met him and knowing nothing of his external life, she claimed intimate knowledge of his inner world. Through months of therapy, she made no effort to confirm even the man's name, let alone what, if anything, had ever happened to him. She demonstrates how dangerous the psychologizing of the 'victim experience' can be in the hands of those who use the technology to manufacture victims and to promote their own theories.

The psychologist Judith Herman wrote in *Trauma and Recovery*: 'The ordinary response to atrocities is to banish them from consciousness . . . Atrocities, however, refuse to be buried . . . Remembering and telling the truth about terrible events *are prerequisites* both for the restoration of the social order and for the healing of individual victims.'[7] Few people recognize the subtle but profound effect of psychologizing inherent in such statements. In these excerpts, which are consistent with the theme of the book, Herman expresses her conviction (theory) that terrible events (specifically sexual and domestic violence) cannot be forgotten, must be remembered and must be talked about.

Psychologizing is not a process exclusive to victims of abuse or violence nor did it originate in the current Psychology Industry. In fact the American philosopher William James, as early as 1900, expressed concern in this regard:

> I hope that Freud and his pupils will push their ideas to their utmost limits, so that we may learn what they are. They can't fail to throw light on human nature, but I confess that he made on me personally the impression of a man *obsessed with fixed ideas*. I

> can make nothing in my own case with his dream theories, and obviously '*symbolism is a most dangerous method*'.[8]

What concerned James was that Freud and his followers would forget that their ideas were theories and instead, would *listen for* material from patients that would support their psychologizing, ignoring any conflicting data. He feared that with their 'obsessed thinking', they would apply fixed and predetermined ideas about people and change their words into a symbolic language. The danger that James foresaw was that they would hear only what they expected to hear and that they would turn the experiences of individuals into a general experience; thus, a patient would become equated with all other patients with 'similar' problems.

This process of applying a theory to turn what people say into a 'deeper', psychologized meaning, turning a unique experience into a general one through the use of abstract concepts, has been pushed to the limits in the interpretation of the experiences of victims, both real and fabricated. The danger which James detected in the psychologists' 'fixed ideas' and 'symbolism' has infiltrated and contaminated the study of 'victims'.

An example, and only one of many possible examples of this process, involves the work of Robert Lifton. A psychiatrist with a psychoanalytic bent, Lifton is a pioneer in the study of victims. He describes himself as a 'psychiatric investigator', having examined those who survived the Nazi death camps, the bombing of Hiroshima and the Vietnam War. He describes his work as 'a form of *re-creation*'.[9] He listens but, by his own admission, he does so believing that 'in contrast to the more immediate involvement of other animals, human beings experience their world by *symbolizing*'.[10] He claims that 'as human beings we know our bodies and our minds *only through what we can imagine*' and that

> to grasp our humanity *we need to structure these images into metaphors and models* . . . In other words, psychologists do not simply interpret or analyze; we also construct; we engage in our own struggles

> around form. We are much concerned with narrative, and we inevitably contribute to the narrative of whatever life we examine.[11]

Lifton approached his subjects with a specific interest in concepts like that of psychic numbing (i.e. the effect of seeing death) and death guilt (i.e. of surviving when others died). He listened to specific ideas and images. From this, he constructed theories to create a model of what he thought went on inside people's minds, in their unconscious.

When his interpretation is placed alongside the words of victims, such as Elie Wiesel, the filtering and distorting effects of psychologizing become apparent. Read how Robert Lifton interprets Wiesel's experiences as described in *Night*, translating the author's words into terms which fit his psychologized 'survivor syndrome' and theory of 'death guilt':

> The survivor of Nazi concentration camps moreover, like the survivor of Hiroshima, carried the burden not only of what he did but what he felt. Thus, Wiesel tells how, as a fifteen-year-old boy, he took tender care of his sick father under the most extreme conditions en route to and within Auschwitz, Buna, and Buchenwald. But when temporarily separated from him he was suddenly horrified at his wish that he not be able to find him: 'If only I could get rid of the dead weight, so that I could use all my strength to struggle for my own survival, and only worry about myself.' And when his father died, he perceived 'in the recess of my weakened conscience,' a feeling close to 'free at last!' He describes feeling both guilty and 'ashamed of myself, ashamed forever;' and the indelibility of the imprint of these events is more forcefully conveyed when he recalls how, shortly after being liberated (and following a severe illness of his own), he looked into a mirror and 'a corpse gazed back at me. The look in his eyes, as they stared into mine, has never left me.'[12]

But does this psychologizing make Wiesel's experience truly more understandable? Years after his ordeal, having returned to Birkenau and Auschwitz, Wiesel spoke of what had happened there not merely in terms of what was going on inside his head but also in terms of what was happening around him. Remembering his father, he said:

> The Russian soldiers could have saved him. But they arrived too late, too late – for us. We had already been marched off to Gleiwitz, and from there, in open cattle cars, to Buchenwald. We were surrounded by corpses; we no longer knew who was alive and who was not. I remember a man – my father – murmuring to himself, or to the icy wind that lashed his face: 'What a pity, what a pity . . .'[13]

Lifton takes these immediate and personal experiences and 're-creates' them according to his psychological theories. In support of his notion of 'death guilt' as part of the victim experience, he writes:

> Sometimes the delayed guilt takes the form of remembered voices of those left to die while one was oneself being rescued – as described by the elderly widow, who was carried to safety in a wheelbarrow by her son and daughter-in-law: 'I heard many voices calling for help, voices calling their father, voices of women and children . . . I couldn't move my body very well, and my son had six children to take care of in addition to me, so, well, we just didn't help people . . . I felt it was a wrong thing not to help them, but we were so much occupied by running away ourselves that we left them . . . Even now I still hear the voices . . .'[14]

Why would one who is earnestly interested in understanding victims reconstruct their experiences filtering out the personal vividness? One explanation may be found in Lifton's writing about his interviews with Hiroshima survivors:

> I was confronted with the brutal details . . . I noticed that my reactions were changing. I was listening to descriptions of the same horrors, but their effect on me lessened. *I concentrated upon recurrent patterns* . . . The experience was an unforgettable demonstration of the psychic closing-off we shall see to be characteristic of all aspects of atomic bomb exposure, even of this kind of exposure to the exposed. It also taught me *the importance of making sense of the event*, of calling upon one's personal and professional resources to give it form, *as means of coping with it.*[15]

Listening to authentic victims has an effect on the listener, an effect which may make listening difficult and create the need to change the experiences into a pattern, a theory that seems to make sense; something with which the psychologist can cope.

It is appropriate for Lifton, as a researcher, to search for patterns in the ways authentic victims handle their experiences. However, it becomes 'a most dangerous method', to quote James, when this search for patterns involves distorting the words spoken and assuming that the pattern fits *all* victims. Lifton did this when he wrote: '*The survivor is one* who has come into contact with death in some bodily or psychic fashion and has remained alive. There are five characteristic themes in the survivor: the death imprint, death guilt, psychic numbing, conflicts around nurturing and contagion, and struggles with meaning or formulation.'[16]

Stated thus, his simplified theory becomes a template that can be easily turned into a rationale for psychological treatment. To the psychologist, a person's lack of emotions or questions about the purpose of life or a sense of grief, all become signs that the individual is or has been a victim. Each person ostensibly is someone whose inner world must be explored in expectation of confirming theories about 'the victim experience'. Listening for themes and patterns, psychologists find them.

Psychoanalysis is not the only arena in which psychologizing occurs. Elizabeth Kubler-Ross studied terminally ill patients and, through her observation and interviews, she developed a theory about the psychological stages that people go through in preparing to die: denial, anger, bargaining, depression, acceptance and hope.[17] It was to be a psychological model that may lead to some descriptive understanding of the experience. However, the Psychology Industry has turned around theories like this one, and those of Lifton and others, creating from them blueprints of psychological processes.

Thus, theories initially intended to expand the understanding of victims, survivors and the dying, become useful to enterprising psychologists. The theories which describe the experience become the basis for determining who is a victim. For example, anyone who claims to be 'out of touch with their feelings' can be said to be numbed and, therefore, to be a victim. The same theories also become the basis for establishing the proper treatment procedure, such as, in the case of someone 'numbed', removing the blocks to intense emotions through uncovering repressed memories. Some theorists make this turn-about easier by being dogmatic, ignoring the victim's actual words in favour of their own theories; others do it by employing apparently magical powers, reading the victim's unconscious, creating and interpreting symbolism.

An unfortunate result of psychologizing is that the personal experiences of victims become the clinical theories through which others are assessed and treated as if they are victims; psychologizing promotes victim-making.

Pathologizing

> *I think we should stop divinizing psychiatry* and *start humanizing it.* To begin with, we must learn to differentiate between what is human in man and what is pathological in him . . . Sigmund Freud, it is true, once wrote that 'The moment one inquires about the sense or value of life, one is sick,' but I rather think that one thereby manifests one's humanness.[18]

Another aspect of victim-making involves looking for and emphasizing the negative, pointing to wounds, scars, weaknesses and lasting effects. Pathologizing the experiences of victims turns their normal feelings into abnormal states and their normal reactions into emotional problems.

Some time after the young woman described in the introduction was abducted and held captive, a newspaper article was written by a reporter who highlighted the brutality of the woman's experience.

The woman quickly wrote a response to the newspaper, expressing her own views on why these graphic and extremely personal details should not have been made available 'for public consumption'. For her, she said, the ordeal was essentially over; she no longer wanted to be 'the victim'. Like the ordeal, being a victim was part of her past; she wanted to live in the present and get on with her life. She pointed out that, as well as ignoring how the article could harm her, the reporter had failed to take a constructive angle to her story: 'For example, why not explore the circumstances that kept the victim alive: How she dealt with the offender and how she kept her will to live in a traumatic situation beyond her control and conception of reality?'[19]

We have become so accustomed to thinking of victims in terms of trauma that it is very difficult to bring ourselves to consider survivors as anything other than psychologically damaged. To do as this woman suggests would be to emphasize her strength over her helplessness. And this is not what the Psychology Industry wants.

Wiesel offers another example of this inclination toward pathologizing in a chapter he wrote entitled 'Trivializing Memory':

> As for philosophers and psychiatrists, some of them have long been *intrigued by simplistic theories* . . . In the course of scholarly colloquia, one sometimes hears more about the guilt of the victims and the psychological problems of the survivors than about the crimes of the killers. Didn't an American novelist recently suggest that the suicide of my friend Primo Levi was nothing but *a bout of depression* that good psychoanalytic treatment could have cured. Thus is the

tragedy of a great writer, a man who never ceased to battle the black angel of Auschwitz, reduced to *a banal nervous breakdown.*[20]

Whether it is to ignore the personal strengths of the individual or the appropriate reactions to the reality of the experience itself, the Psychology Industry tends to turn authentic victims into damaged people. As one psychologist said about 'the camp experience': 'To one degree or another they [the prisoners] *all stifled* their true feelings, they *all denied* the dictates of conscience and social feeling in hope of survival, and they were *all warped and distorted* as a result.'[21]

We can wonder why this belief that victims are psychologically damaged people exists, or, as Des Pres puts it: 'Why . . . do we insist that survivors did not really survive: that . . . their spirit was destroyed beyond salvaging?'[22]

The answer to this lies, at least in part, in the writings of those who claim to understand 'the victim experience'.

One of the most influential is Bruno Bettelheim, whose concept of 'survivorship' consists of the classic traumatic cause and pathological effect:

(1) the original trauma which, in the context of the Holocaust, is '*the personality-disintegrating impact* of being imprisoned in a German concentration camp which completely destroyed one's social existence by depriving one of all previous support systems such as family, friends, position in life, while at the same time subjecting one to utter terrorization and degradation through the severest mistreatment and omnipresent, inescapable, immediate threat to one's life'; and

(2) 'the *life-long aftereffects* of such trauma, which seem to require very special forms of mastery if one is not to succumb to them.'[23]

Claiming to have been trained as a psychologist in Vienna, Bettelheim derived much of his authority from his limited experience as a prisoner in Dachau and Buchenwald early in the war (1938–39). Released before these camps became the scenes of mass extermination, which Wiesel and others lived to describe, Bettelheim moved to America, where he wrote an academic article in which he presented his 'clinical observations' of his fellow prisoners. Published in

1943, it gave Bettelheim an early position of authority on victims, a position enhanced by his public image as both a psychologist and a survivor.[24] It is clear from this article and his subsequent writings that, even while a prisoner, he assumed the role of a psychologist looking for and finding pathology in others.

While other survivors talked of keeping the rituals of their Jewish religion or of the importance of family and relationships to their survival, Bettelheim described himself as 'a student of psychoanalysis and a follower of Freud' who had his own 'idiosyncratic' way of surviving by falling back on his 'faith' in psychoanalysis.[25]

From the outset, Bettelheim saw his fellow prisoners as abnormal people. In his initial 1943 paper, he distanced himself from them by referring to himself as 'the author', 'the observer', 'the thinker', even the 'normal one':

> The author saw his fellow prisoners acting in most peculiar ways, although he had every reason to assume that they, too, had been normal persons before being imprisoned: Now they suddenly appeared to be *pathological* liars, to be unable to restrain their emotional outbursts, be they of anger or despair, to be unable to make objective evaluations . . .[26]

Bettelheim proceeded to develop his theories by psychologizing and pathologizing survivors. For instance, he suggested three alternative responses to being a victim:

> The most destructive of these three possible responses was to unconsciously conclude that the reintegration of one's personality was impossible, pointless, or both . . . Their state of mind is similar to that of an individual *suffering from a depressive or paranoid psychiatric disturbance* . . .
>
> There were other survivors – and they may well be the majority . . . Survivors who deny that their camp experience has demolished their integration, who *repress guilt* and sense that they ought to live up to some special obligation, often do quite well in life, as

far as appearances go. But emotionally they are depleted because much of their vital energy goes into *keeping denial and repression going*, and because they can no longer trust their inner integration to offer them security, should it again be put to the test for it failed once before. So, while these survivors are relatively symptom free, their life is in some essential respects, deep down, full of inner insecurity . . .

Finally, there is the group of survivors who concluded from their experience that only a better integration would permit them to live as well as they could with the aftereffects of their concentration camp experience . . . *A precondition for a new integration is acceptance of how severely one has been traumatized, and of what the nature of the trauma has been.*[27]

Thus Bettelheim managed to make even those who neither reported nor demonstrated any pathology look sick; to ignore what the majority of victims were saying, and to conclude that:

(1) All victims are psychologically damaged.
(2) All survivors need psychological treatment.

These conclusions turn all victims into potential patients. The Psychology Industry and the public have come to know and accept Bettelheim's conclusions, now popularized, as 'clinical truths'. While his ideas are not always attributed to him, 'His version is *the* version'[28] not only for interpreting the experiences of concentration-camp survivors but for describing the experiences of other survivors. His concept of 'survivorship' has been extrapolated to fit any and all victims, including manufactured ones.

As Bettelheim, with an air of psychological superiority, viewed all his fellow prisoners as psychologically damaged, suffering 'life-long aftereffects', so too does the Psychology Industry now view all people who have experienced any 'traumatic event' (real or imaginary) as suffering long-term psychopathology. As he considered the options for concentration-camp survivors to be either a lifetime of denial,

Pathologizing

VICTIMS ==> ABNORMAL

these terms "normal/abnormal"
are then used to turn

VICTIMS <== ABNORMAL <== PEOPLE

repression and underlying insecurity or possible new integration through psychotherapy, so too do psychologists present these two options to 'victims': to be 'in denial' or be 'in therapy'. For Bettelheim, the preferable solution was a process of 'working through', beginning with an acceptance of the trauma and its terrible impact. For psychologists, it is a similar process of confronting the memory and understanding its devastating effects. But the Psychology Industry doesn't stop at assessing pathology in all victims. It goes further by identifying pathology in everyone, making everyone a victim. To do this it plays with the notion of 'normal'.

Measurement of human qualities was the original basis on which psychology became distinct from both philosophy and medicine and came to be recognized as a science. It grew as a profession as its measuring devices were applied in education, industry and the military. Its tests assessed the normal range of intelligence; measured the normal abilities for workers; and determined the normal personality for soldiers.

To create these tests, psychologists determined what 'normal' was by measuring the characteristics of thousands of people and then calculating an average and a normal range. In the same way that a normal range of temperature or rainfall can be calculated, so a normal range of intelligence, ability or behaviour could be established.

But psychologists have twisted this concept of 'normal'. Instead of referring to something quantitative and objective, it now refers to something qualitative and subjective. The original concept of 'normal' as average has been replaced by the psychological one involving pathology. No longer does 'normal' have to do with the common experience of people, for psychologists have made normal such a narrow range that most people today are, by some definition or another, abnormal. Today 'normal' is how psychologists think the world should be: how families should function, how couples ought to 'enjoy intimacy', how one ought to 'resolve conflicts'. It portrays the image of a psychological utopia and defines all those without perfect lives as 'victims'. For if they are not 'normal' by psychology's standard, then something is wrong; they have pathology and, according to the Psychology Industry, their pathology is most likely the result of having been a victim. Those who grew up in 'dysfunctional families' become 'adult children of alcoholics'; those who have less than ideal marriages evidence past 'abuse'; those who have less than ideal lives must find 'the hidden cause'.

One can then better understand the protest of the young woman when she challenges the reporter who failed to say anything about her strengths, her skills, her ability to survive. In this pathologizing world in which she is trying to get on with her life, only her negative feelings, her weaknesses and her problems were seen to count; 'once a victim, always a victim'.

Bettelheim is largely responsible for this tendency to pathologize the victim experience. Throughout his writings, he:

1) exhibited a paternalistic concern, observing his companion prisoners from a personally distanced and psychoanalytically detached perspective. In describing his early experience at Dachau, he wrote:

> While swapping tales that morning, it suddenly flashed through my mind, this is driving me crazy . . . That was when I decided that rather than be taken in by such rumours I would try to understand what was psychologically behind them . . . While some prisoners were reticent, most were more than willing to talk about themselves, because to find someone interested in them and their problems *helped their badly shaken self esteem.*[29]

2) based his conclusions on his own, very limited concentration-camp experience. In doing so, he assumed a paradoxical approach, distancing himself from the other *prisoners* (they were abnormal, he was normal) but then equating all other *survivors* to himself when he spoke of the need to engage in a lifelong psychological struggle to cope.

3) infantilized victims, seeing them as 'incompetent children', incapable of doing things for themselves and viewing the guards as harsh father figures. For example, he wrote: 'prisoners were often mistreated in ways that a cruel and domineering father might use against helpless children.'[30]

4) thought that the trauma made it impossible to have healthy personal and social relationships. In contrast to other survivors' reports, he stated that they 'were not real friends; they were companions at work, and more often in misery. But while misery loves company, it does not make for friendship. Genuine attachments just do not grow in a barren field of experience nourished only by emotions of frustration and despair . . .'[31]

5) described all prisoners in negative ('sick') terms, thus denying the strong coping behaviours of some prisoners such as those who worked in the underground while in camps.

6) considered *all* survivors to be in need of help in their long-term struggle to deal with their problems. Not only did Bettelheim see the need for psychotherapy; he saw that 'the survivor's new integration will be . . . more meaningful than that of many a person who has been spared subjection to an extreme experience.'[32] Thus he was one of the first of the modern-day breed of psychologist to make the 'victim's' experience seem special, bestowing on victims a sense of importance, and describing psychotherapy as a 'heroic journey'.

These flaws:

- assuming a paternalistic attitude,
- using their own limited and sometimes unrelated experiences,

- treating other people as children,
- pathologizing relationships,
- ignoring personal strengths of individuals,
- identifying the need for psychological treatment

characterize the approach of the Psychology Industry as it manufactures victims.

Bettelheim also developed a further pathologized abstraction, one now embraced by the Psychology Industry, by arguing that verbal threats in the concentration camps were *more* damaging than physical assaults. He wrote:

> Even the cruellest parent threatens physical punishment much more often than he actually inflicts it, so childlike feelings of helplessness were created much more effectively by the constant threat of beatings than by actual torture. During a real beating one could, for example, take some pride in suffering manfully, in not giving the foreman or guard the satisfaction of grovelling before him, etc. No such emotional protection was possible against the mere threat.[33]

Thus the thought becomes more powerful than the act; the word more damaging than the deed; the fantasy more real than the fact. Such was the personal philosophy of Bettelheim. As Richard Pollak writes in his recent devastating biography, Bettelheim embraced a philosophy that 'held, generally, that because life had no real purpose it was made livable only by pretending through fictions that it did'.[34] His own life, on examination, is an example of such a work of fiction. He was never trained as a psychologist or a psychoanalyst; he exaggerated his 'studies' of concentration-camp life; and his 'cures' of autistic children were not verifiable. As Lehman-Haupt writes: 'Bettelheim seems to have re-enacted the archetypal American success story of inventing a false past, concocting a new formula for snake oil, and selling it to the public with flummery.'[35]

Despite the exposed fraud, the Psychology Industry still accepts his approach by which all victims become patients; the stage remains set for all the world to become a victim.

Generalizing: The Dangerous 'Slippery Slope'

A trauma is a trauma is a trauma![36]

During the Iran hostage crisis of the late 1970s, a group of mental-health professionals met regularly to plan the best way to offer the psychological help which, it was assumed, the hostages would need once they were released. From the start, the members of the group admitted that, as hard as they tried, they found it difficult to put themselves into the hostages' place – 'to feel deep in our guts, what their experience of captivity might actually be like.' One member of the group describes how they managed to solve this problem:

> A member of our group asked us to think: Were our lives really so far removed from those of the hostages? How many of us had cause to *regard ourselves as victims*?
>
> As it turned out, nearly all of us had recently *felt threatened or exploited*. The actual episodes reported by the group members differed widely. One social worker had been the *victim of a break-in*. A psychologist *had lost* his younger sister to leukaemia. And a psychiatrist had learned of his wife's *plans to leave* him. The result of our collective realization was dramatic. We felt *a powerful surge of empathy* toward the 52 captives, held for over a year, whom we would soon be welcoming back.[37]

Notice the ease with which the group slipped from grappling with the complex question they raised to accepting the simplistic solution that they all knew how the hostages felt because they had felt that way too. Having accepted the suggestion that they could regard themselves as victims, they began to slide into generalizations. They searched inside themselves for feelings of threat and exploitation, slipping into their own experiences and losing sight of those of the hostages. Quickly, they became involved in their own issues, talking excitedly about their own experiences of break-ins, death and divorce. Eventually, drawing 'dramatic' comparisons between their lives and those of the hostages, they concluded that they shared the experience and the effects.

They demonstrate a bizarre form of 'psycho-thinking' which can be called 'slippery-slope logic'. On this slippery slope, people, like those in the group, begin with a rational thought and then, in gradual stages, slide into irrational conclusions, always believing that each thought along the way makes sense. In what seems like a mental toboggan ride, they slide down backwards, not noticing their descent or bothering to compare where they land at the bottom of the hill with where they began at the top.

Generalizing
"the slippery slope"

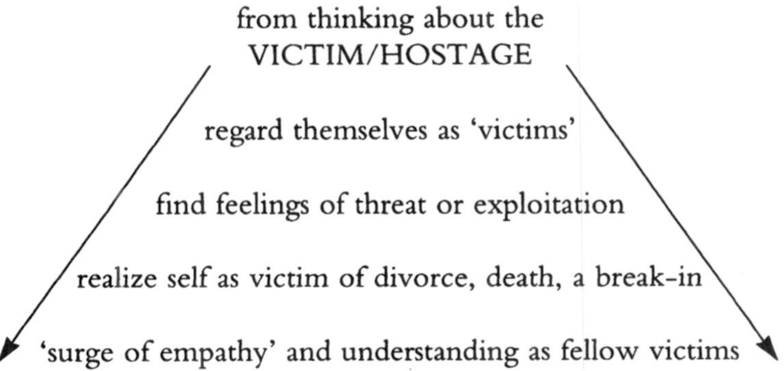

A group of professionals managed to conclude that they knew how captives being held in an Iranian prison would feel once they were released. They reached this point by thinking about how they might see themselves as victims. Not one individual, it seems, questioned whether they could, in fact, legitimately regard themselves as victims. In the spirit of generalizing, they convinced themselves that they too were victims and placed themselves, along with the hostages, in a general survivor category. They ceased grappling with the insurmountable challenge of putting themselves into the hostages' place. Sitting in a comfortable room, exchanging stories from their own lives, they began to imagine deep in their guts what it felt like to be a victim and then imagined that it was the same as being held captive in an Iranian prison.

Could they have managed as easily to identify with Holocaust or Hiroshima survivors? Probably. Consider this example, taken from Lifton's writings:

> It is precisely this kind of death guilt, rather than external events in themselves, which survivors of Nazi camps and Hiroshima refer to when they speak of their 'living hell.' And from these extreme experiences we come to realize that no one's emotions about death and survival are ever experienced entirely as individual matters; that images of dying are bound up with inner questions about who and what will survive, and images of surviving with who (and what) has died in one's place.
>
> Analogous patterns of guilt over survival priority have been observed in lesser disasters, and in relationship to dying patients. Again, the doctor attending these patients experiences the emotions of a survivor and 'must contend with the guilt evoked by the questioning glance of the dying, with the unspoken question, 'Why should I die while you live?'[38]

In this case, on the slope made slippery through the psychologized concept of death guilt, Lifton begins with the experience of a prisoner watching another die and ends up equating that with a physician attending a dying patient.

With this logic, one could continue the slide into the conclusion that all physicians suffer from 'survivor syndrome'. To take this a slide further, anyone and everyone who has ever seen anyone die or known anyone who has died, might then wonder about death and survival. Ipso facto, all adults do, or one day will, suffer from 'survivor syndrome'.

With Lifton, the possibility for 'slippery-slope logic' can be seen in the slide from surviving the Holocaust:

to
surviving while others were victims
to
surviving while patients die
to
surviving while anyone dies.

Thus, all of us have something in common with death-camp survivors: we have all survived someone else's death.

Lifton himself doesn't take it quite this far but he begins the descent. And others do slide all the way to the bottom. They begin with the concept of victim which, in the context of external events, does have real meaning, and they accept the psychologized, pathologized understanding which makes it an idea, an image, a stereotype. Then they slide backwards into other popularized words and ideas, such as 'stress' and 'grief', and end up at the bottom of the slope, with everything meaning 'victim', and 'victim' not meaning anything at all.

Along with psychologizing and pathologizing, 'generalizing', as practised by the Psychology Industry, becomes another aspect of manufacturing victims.

In the Introduction, a psychologist was quoted as saying that whether the crime was murder or rape, or a purse snatched or a pocket picked, the internal injury was the same. Below, one of the 'victims' cited in his book describes their experience:

> You feel stripped naked. You feel as if someone has exposed you totally . . . You're powerless . . . You're powerless. Violation is an adult way to explain that, but it isn't an adult response. It's reminiscent of the kind of helplessness that goes back to early childhood. And I think that's what makes it so crucially painful. Because you can't fight back.[39]

These are the thoughts of the 'victim of a purse snatching'. They demonstrate 'generalizing', showing how people come to experience events when they follow the scripts provided by the Psychology Industry. A pocket picked becomes as emotionally injurious as a rape, angry words become as abusive as a physical attack. Psychologists define the psychological importance of events ('it's just as bad as . . .') and ignore the nature of the external events. Years ago, children used to have a playground chant: 'Sticks and stones may break my bones but names'll never hurt me.' They knew the differences between insults and assaults. But today the Psychology Industry is telling everyone that an angry word hurts like a bullet. With psychologists' help, everyone can share the experiences of victims and by so doing, can come to see themselves as victims.

A Victim Does Not a Patient Make

> *Attempts to interpret the survivors' experience – to see it in terms other than its own – have done more harm than good.*[40]

Julius Segal, a psychologist who has worked with returned prisoners of war, hostages, Holocaust survivors, refugees and others who have experienced extreme traumas, provided the example above of the group preparing to treat the hostages. As he stated:

> . . . according to popular expectations, [the hostages] should have become victims of lifelong emotional problems. For months prior to [their] release, pundits and professionals alike offered dire predictions of the outcome of our captives in Teheran. Unhealable scars would blemish their psyches, we were told, and they would remain emotional and physical wrecks for the rest of their lives. One psychologist announced her mournful prognoses on national television: '. . . permanent problems in interpersonal relationships . . . permanent coordination difficulties . . . permanent damage to memory.'[41]

Bettelheim made similar predictions for survivors of the Nazi extermination camps:

> . . . the assumption that these prisoners developed states of mind similar to those observed in psychotic persons seems borne out by the behaviour of former prisoners of extermination camps after their liberation. In some persons the symptoms appeared more severe, in others less so; some showed that their symptoms were reversible, others not . . . Some were still suffering from delusions of persecution, others suffered from delusions of grandeur. The latter were the counterpart of guilt feelings for having been spared while parents or siblings had all perished. They were trying to justify and explain their own survival by delusionally inflating their importance. It also enabled them to compensate for the extreme damage done to their narcissism by the experience they had undergone.[42]

These expectations, and similarly negative ones, exist for all victims no matter what the traumatic event is that they experienced. It would seem that a victim does a patient make. However, Segal continued on from the paragraph above by stating: 'No such forecasts have been realized . . . the hostages emerged to freedom *without lingering symptoms*: no disabling anxiety or depression, no lacerating guilt, no insuperable problems readapting to the world.'[43]

So, despite experiences of brutal interrogations, isolation, threats of execution, and suffering from malnutrition and dysentery, they managed to resume normal living without the anticipated psychological problems. Again, as Segal wrote: 'This case is not unique. For over thirty years, I have studied victims of overwhelming stress . . . repeatedly, I have been inspired by the countless cases that run counter to "experts" predictions.'[44]

There are, in fact, many studies which show the strength and adaptability of survivors. One study of Holocaust survivors draws attention to 'the magnificent ability of human beings to rebuild shattered lives, careers, and families, even as they wrestle with the bitterest of memories'.[45] In another, Anton Antonovsky, studying concentration-camp survivors, writes of his fascination that 'a not-inconsiderable number of concentration camp survivors were found to be well-adapted . . . what, we must ask, has given these women the strength, despite their experiences, to maintain what would seem to be the capacity not only to function well, but even to be happy.'[46] Peter Suedfeld, through laboratory experiments on restricted stimulation, field studies in polar stations, archival analyses of decision-making under stress, and interviews with Holocaust survivors, makes a strong argument for the fortitude and resilience of human beings in the face of severe situations.[47]

When survivors' experiences are examined by researchers who are not advocates of a particular theory, there are few abstractions found to support themes such as Lifton's 'death guilt' or Bettelheim's pathologized view of survivors. For instance, Sylvia Rothchild, after listening to hundreds of interviews with survivors, commented: 'Expecting them to be sad, even morbid, I wasn't prepared for the flashes of exhilaration, for the strength and pride of life-obsessed people who had lived through the worst of times . . .'[48] She noted that when asked how they have lived after their experiences, the responses were richly varied but specific and concrete:

> A survivor from Sobibor says he lives but has no appetite for life: 'I have deep feelings for other survivors but basically I believe most people are rotten.' A woman who escaped with him has another nature. 'I'm happy and content,' she says. 'I like my life and my self . . .' Survivors respond differently to violence. 'If somebody hits you with a rock,' says Elizabeth Mermelstein, 'throw him back a piece of bread.' A survivor of Sobibor says: 'Only fighting back can give you honour and respect.'[49]

So how is it that the popular belief is one of deep damage and long-term distress? Why do we believe that victims are so weakened by their experience that they can never recover unless they cease to deny the devastating effects of 'the trauma', uncover it, face it, confront it and go through the required psychological healing process? Later chapters will show that it is in a large part due to the influence of those who benefit from this prediction. As the psychologist Norman Garmezy from the University of Minnesota said: 'our mental health practitioners and researchers are predisposed by interest, investment, and training in seeing deviance, psychopathology, and weakness wherever they look.'[50]

The horrific suffering that some victims bear cannot be trivialized or denied, nor can it be implied that people never carry scars. There are authentic victims and some of these people do have trouble coping with life because of what happened to them. It must be fully acknowledged that some victims need help in living with the effects of their experience, and as Bettelheim says: 'some will get better and some will not.' What is questionable is the stereotyping of all victims into a common patient image and the use of that image to benefit the Psychology Industry.

As Segal discovered, and as astute observers find repeatedly, people manifest remarkable resilience. The Psychology Industry, its beliefs and practices, have been largely responsible for the creation of a world in which people live in fear that they will crumble. It repeatedly confirms the fear which most have when listening to the story of someone like Wiesel or the young rape victim that 'if that happened to me I couldn't cope' and it encourages the response: 'I can't get over it' even to events which pale in comparison.

The idea has been planted in the heads of most people that if they falter at all, doubt themselves at all, ever fear or ever fail, they lack 'the inner strength', 'the self-esteem', 'the power' to deal with their own lives. They believe that their 'egos have been tattered', their 'energy has been depleted' and, seeing themselves as 'victims', they become users of the Psychology Industry.

2
Fabricated Victims

As our fifteenth-century forebears were obsessed with the creation of saints and our nineteenth-century ancestors with the creation of heroes, from Christopher Columbus to George Washington, so are we with the recognition, praise and, when necessary, the manufacture of victims.

Robert Hughes

The young woman abducted and raped, the accident victim whose life was shattered, Elie Wiesel, the Iranian student, the hostages – not one of these people would have chosen to have happen to them what happened. As Des Pres points out, 'survivors do not choose their fate and would escape if they could.'[1] So, why, when authentic victims would escape if they could, are people today allowing themselves to be categorized as victims?

Being a real victim involves pain, injury and loss. In contrast, becoming a fabricated victim entails none of these obvious costs. Rather, it amounts to being reassured that the worst thing that can happen has already occurred and that help is on the way. The Psychology Industry sells the idea that once identified as a victim, one can anticipate relief and healing and 'happily-ever-after' endings. One self-described abuse victim writes:

> From a destitute addict to a healthy, happy participant in life, I have found my Prince Charming, and maybe someday we'll even

> have a castle. It isn't always easy but, with support, I've at least gained the courage to try. Every fairy tale I ever read as a kid had a happy ending, and I'll be damned if mine doesn't too.[2]

Recognition as a victim provides the starting point. It identifies the client as the central character and the psychologist as the guide in some heroic journey, the modern-day quest for innocence and fulfilment. Becoming a fabricated victim isn't about endings and losses so much as it is about beginnings and gains.

What all fabricated victims have in common is not some extraordinary experience but rather the expectation of a future made brighter by virtue of victim status. Fabricated victims are given permission to lead psychologized lives, where guilt and shame are banished and responsibilities are diminished. Meanwhile, those unidentified by the Psychology Industry must go on with their lives complete with disappointments, failures, self-doubts, embarrassing moments, regrets, sicknesses, debts, and even sins to be confessed and crimes for which to be punished.

People adopt this status for many reasons. There are *synthetic victims*: the ordinary, often quite normal people who are brought under the Psychology Industry's pervasive influence. Receptive, suggestible or momentarily vulnerable, these are the people who come to accept as factual some revised, reinterpreted or fictionalized version of their lives.

There are *contrived victims*: the people who have been diagnosed with medical problems to which the Psychology Industry attributes a psychological cause, solution or need. Sick, suffering and often desperate, these people are easily swayed by misinformation and false hopes.

Then there are *counterfeit victims*: the people who intentionally lie and for whom psychologists become paid accomplices. They knowingly make up stories, feign symptoms, play sick or injured in order to escape blame, avoid punishment, find an excuse, get even with someone, extort money or gain attention.

Synthetic Victims

> *Victimism debilitates its practitioners by trapping them in a world of oppressive demons that they cannot, by definition, control.*[3]

'They tell you that everything you knew for twenty, thirty, forty years was wrong. Your parents, whom you trusted, the values they instilled in you as a child. You're told they are all garbage . . . Anything you say can be and will be misinterpreted. There is no way around it.'[4]

This is how Lynn Gondolf describes the Psychology Industry as it turns people into victims. She had entered therapy hoping to find a solution to her chronic eating disorder. At the beginning, she told her psychologist about being raped by an uncle. She had always remembered clearly what had happened: 'that wasn't anything I'd forgotten or ever would forget.' And she told her therapist that she could understand that there might be some connection to her problems since her uncle had always given her a dollar for candy after each incident. But the psychologist was not satisfied that she was expressing 'enough' emotion and insisted that there must be more buried somewhere deep in her unconscious.

He interpreted her dreams and her drawings, and had her do automatic writing during hypnosis, as he led her to search for hidden signs that other members of her family had abused her as well. He insisted that she attend a group of women for the purpose of remembering more about what had been done to them. 'They wanted us to talk about experiences very explicitly in front of the others and get into a rage,' she reports. 'It gets contagious. This one says she remembers something, then this one, then this one. The stories got grosser and grosser and you had a tiny roomful of girls screaming and raging and bawling. If you didn't have memories, you didn't get any attention. I can dream stuff up, sure . . .' Eventually, when Gondolf began to 'remember' episodes of her father raping her, the psychologist called in her brother and sisters, and told them that she'd probably kill herself unless they supported her in these allegations.

A year later, Gondolf had accused her father of sexually abusing her, been diagnosed with various depressive disorders, gone from taking no medication to using a mixture of eight different drugs, lost her job, and become entirely dependent on her psychologist. By the time her insurance money ran out, she had hit rock bottom. Her psychologist then decided to end treatment, attributing her failure to her resistance and noncompliance. He tried to have her committed to a state institution but she sought treatment to withdraw from the medication and 'slowly began to learn how to live again, how to work things out by myself'. She came to realize that her father 'hadn't done a thing'.

It took two years for Gondolf to function normally again. As she describes it, 'I'd believe all this stuff . . . and you suffer all the psychological trauma as if it all really had gone on.' Gondolf publicly stated that her father was innocent of all the allegations she had made and she became one of the first synthetic victims to talk openly about the devastating effects of the Psychology Industry.

With the current controversy over 'false memories' sparked by such personal accounts, the idea of a false or fabricated victim is most likely to bring to mind someone who has discovered that their memories of abuse are false. There is a growing number of such individuals who claim that they were persuaded by psychologists into accepting they were victims of trauma, only later to discover that what they had come to believe in therapy was not true. With their stories appearing in popular magazines, they have drawn the public's attention to the Psychology Industry's business of manufacturing synthetic victims.

> **Synthetic**: (adj), [Gk synthetikos, of composition] 1. produced artificially, man-made; 2. devised, arranged, or fabricated for special situations to imitate or replace usual realities.
>
> *Webster's Dictionary*

While recovered-memory cases may be the best known, the term 'synthetic victim' has a much broader scope, identifying not only those people turned into 'false memory' victims but also those who have been turned into other types of synthetic victims through tactics including:

'false interpreting' – the application of specific theories and particular therapies,
'false naming' – the fraudulent assignment of diagnoses, labels and explanatory terms,
'false remembering' – the search for traumatic events, their deeper meaning and their casual nature.

Two prominent themes of the Psychology Industry relying on these tactics are:

Trauma: the notion that for every here-and-now problem, there must be a dramatic there-and-then cause; that some event in the past, as far back in time as infancy, was so disturbing that it continues to affect thoughts, feelings and actions.

and

Addiction: the idea that undesirable behaviours are due to something beyond personal control. The traditional model is alcoholism as a 'disease', but numerous variations have developed, often with attribution to current stress or previous trauma.

Whichever theme or blending of themes is applied, the result is that personal problems are seen as 'damage' due to an external cause.

False Interpreting

Alice laughed. 'There's no use trying,' she said: 'One can't *believe impossible things.'*
'I daresay you haven't had much practice,' said the

> *Queen. 'When I was your age, I always did it for half-an-hour a day. Why, sometimes I've believed as many as six impossible things before breakfast.'*[5]

It would seem that a human tendency exists to assume, when two things happen together, that one causes the other. For instance, since paedophiles often collect child pornography, it is commonly accepted that pornography breeds the violation of children. Similarly, it is a popular assumption that verbal insults lead to physical assaults and that negative emotions cause cancer.

But to assume causation can be misleading. 'For example, there is a high correlation between the consumption of diet soft drinks and obesity. Does this mean that artificial sweeteners cause people to become overweight?'[6] Acceptance of comparable false causations lead to a variety of false interpretations on which the Psychology Industry thrives. Bed-wetting has been connected with abuse; even disliking tapioca pudding has been identified as a sign of repressed memories of childhood sexual abuse.[7]

A psychologist, Edith Fiore, illustrates how such connections are expressed:

> Symptoms and problems whose roots were traced to past lives cover a broad spectrum. For example, I now find that almost all patients with chronic weight excess of ten pounds or more have had a lifetime in which they either starved to death or suffered food deprivation for long periods . . . Many of my patients have discovered that the causes of their phobias, fears, and even aversions were rooted in some traumatic event of a previous lifetime.[8]

Of the thousands who read her bestseller, *You Have Been Here Before*, many connect their problems of being overweight or fearful to past life experiences and seek out 'past-life' therapists.

Favouring confirmation over denial, support over doubt, certainty over questioning, contributes to the acceptance of causal connections between whatever problem a person has and whatever cause a psychologist might suggest. As far-fetched as some Psychology Industry explanations sound, there are thousands of people who have become convinced of past-life experiences and, more recently, of UFO abductions and encounters with satanists. The tendency to make and accept causal connections lies at the base of the Psychology Industry's manufacturing of victims through 'false interpretations'. Psychologists' beliefs in the importance of specific symptoms or particular theories can be so strong that they lead to 'illusionary correlations'. What they think they know is often only a partial or fabricated truth based on their perceptions. And what they call reality is a simple interpretation maintained by further misperceptions and the support of others who share their view of reality.

False interpreting is the essential ingredient in the manufacture of synthetic victims; it places the psychologist's beliefs above the client's problems. For the client, this leads to getting 'the therapist's particular brand of psychotherapy, addressing the problem areas that the therapist finds significant. The form of treatment, then, is determined by the therapist's habitual approach and not by the nature of the problem that the patient brings in.'[9]

While the more bizarre of these are being looked upon with progressively more scepticism, those which seem more realistic remain unquestioned. For instance, Schaef claims a high ground of knowledge which she believes is 'beyond therapy, beyond science'. She states: 'Many of the categories found in the *DSM-III* [*Diagnostic and Statistical Manual*] fit much more readily under the rubric of addiction and co-dependence, and working with them with the tools of the Twelve-Step program and "the deep process work" not only was cheaper and easier, it was more effective.'[10] In other words most, if not all, client problems fit her beliefs and practice. And consider Bass and Davis, who believe that almost one quarter of all children are sexually abused before they turn eighteen. They state: 'The long-term effects of child sexual abuse can be so pervasive that it's sometimes hard to pinpoint exactly how the abuse affected you. It permeates everything: your sense of self, your intimate relationships, your sexuality, your parenting, your work life, even your sanity.'[11]

False interpretations have their most profound effect when they are expressed as subtle suggestions. Pittman confesses that while psychologists 'are trained to pretend that we have no value systems at all', in fact, 'psychotherapy involves applying the value system of the therapist to the dilemmas of the clients.'[12] While clients are warned to avoid therapists who make blatant value-laden statements, these same people who issue the warnings are often the ones who couch their interpretations in subtler forms that suggest possibilities and imply likelihoods.

False interpretations can be seen in the statements of psychologists who seem highly professional, respectable and even rational. For instance:

> We all suffer from 'aftershock,' maybe less violently but still at a price we shouldn't have to pay. In fact, aftershock is the disease of today.[13]

> More than half of all women are survivors of childhood sexual trauma . . . it does not have to involve touch . . . incest can occur through words, sounds, or even exposure of the child to sights or acts that are sexual but do not involve her.[14]

> Leavetaking is the universal experience. From birth to death we face a continuum of partings . . . The trauma associated with leavetaking takes various forms. The individual may become mildly or deeply neurotic or even psychotic. There may be depression (sometimes interspersed with euphoria), anger, anxiety, guilt. A person scarred by a parting may drink heavily, worry in excess, become promiscuous. There are other effects: for example, a mother may get fat after her children leave home. Her obesity is an attempt to deny the fact of leavetaking.[15]

All interpretive paths lead to the same core belief; that is, the person is not in control, is damaged internally and someone else is to blame. Laura Pasley, who entered therapy because of an eating disorder, describes how her psychologist, based on his false interpretations, had her believing a long list of 'impossible things' including that her own mother had been trying to kill her for years:

> If Mama bought us groceries and any of them were easily ingested 'binge foods', [my therapist] said it was to kill me. At one point, I took some badly needed groceries back to her, threw the bag and asked if she was trying to kill me because there were some cookies and chips in the bag . . .[16]

Virtually any experience can be reshaped to fit and any attempt a person makes to question false interpretations can be swept aside. Fiore, the past-lives psychologist, describes the case of a young woman who had sought help to overcome a snake phobia.

> After combing back through her life under hypnosis and finding nothing to explain her fears . . . I asked her if she had had an encounter with snakes before she was born. She saw herself as a fifteen-year-old Aztec girl in front of a pyramid watching priests dancing with poisonous snakes in their mouths. She trembled with emotion and reported the bizarre rites in vivid detail.

When the woman became distressed and said: 'I don't believe all that stuff,' Fiore's response was: 'Here is a person who definitely rejected reincarnation, but who had just relived a lifetime that took place four hundred years ago.'[17]

In another instance involving multiple personalities, an angry former patient confronted her psychologist: 'Don't you think it is odd that no one is getting better and that everyone wants to cut and kill themselves after they get into therapy with you?' Deflecting the question in favour of a false interpretation, he responded by asking: 'Which personality am I talking to now?'[18]

These responses illustrate the more obvious attempts to support false interpretation. But psychologists across North America, not only in therapy sessions and popular books but also in professional journals and conferences, on television and in courtrooms, are giving false interpretations, supported by false assumptions and connections. Because they sound reasonable, people accept them, incorporate them in their thinking and apply them to their own lives. The most dangerous of these are the ones which have gone mainstream, influencing people who would not consider themselves 'users' to re-interpret situations and feelings. A sampling of the everyday Psychology Industry interpretations which are so familiar and so universally accepted that they are leading not only individuals but society to false conclusions include:

- People often overeat because they're unhappy. What are you unhappy about?
- Some relationships are toxic and, like anything harmful, must be ended. You owe it to yourself to weed out the toxic ones.
- Spanking a child is like teaching someone that assault is OK.
- Low self-esteem can lead to shopping binges and an entire loss of control over spending.

False Remembering

> *Repressed memories of sexual abuse and satanic abuse are the favorites among therapists. All the elements of a good soap opera are there – sex, drama and money.*[19]

Among the clearest examples of the pernicious influence of the Psychology Industry are cases which involve the rewriting of personal histories in such a way that events which never happened come to be accepted as historical facts. Called by some 'the quackery of the twentieth-century'[20] and 'the black eye of psychology',[21] recovered memory therapy (RMT) is the segment of the Psychology Industry which has already come under public and professional scrutiny.

RMT, or 'memory work' as it is often called, is based on the fixed belief that psychological problems are caused by traumas, most likely sexual and most often experienced in childhood, and that any inability to remember them fully is due to 'denial' and 'repression'. The Psychology Industry contends that the key to eliminating their impact lies in recovering and re-experiencing the memories. 'The patient must reconstruct not only what happened but also what she felt,' states Herman; 'the recitation of facts without the accompanying emotions is a sterile exercise, without therapeutic effect.'[22]

Most people assume that events are either remembered or forgotten and find it difficult to understand how memories can exist in this netherland of 'repression'. To explain this, Alice Miller writes that abused children 'will not remember the torments to which they were exposed, because those torments, together with the needs related to them, have all been repressed: that is, completely banished from consciousness . . . And later, as adults, they have forgotten such experiences, or at least the memory [is] not vivid enough to cause them to speak of them.'[23]

Proponents of this approach rely on false interpretations, along with leading suggestions and supportive encouragement, to convince people that there may be things in their past which they have forgotten and that 'repressed memories' are the cause of their problems. Since virtually everyone has a span of time they can't remember clearly, and recalls relatively little from early childhood, a psychologist probing these gaps and connecting them with some hidden trauma can make people receptive to the idea. 'If you can't remember what happened that summer, perhaps something happened that you won't want to remember' or 'If you can't remember precisely how it all happened, perhaps we need to go over it in your mind until it becomes clear.' Even people who previously had no concept of being victims can begin to think it possible. When the psychologist explains it in technical terms, it can seem to make sense: 'You have a problem which you have described to me but you can look at it only on the surface. I can help you look at it below the surface and find the source of what is wrong. Then we can fix it.'

Once people are convinced of the possible existence of hidden memories, they can accept that the goal of therapy is to uncover them, perhaps through hypnosis or guided imagery sessions in which scenarios are suggested or events imagined. At other times, psychologists rely on dreams, drawings or family photographs to stimulate ideas and thoughts which can then be rehearsed until they become accepted as memories. In cases where memories already exist, the goal becomes one of reviewing and *revising the memories* until they are experienced with stronger emotion and new meaning.

In 1968, the psychiatrist Herbert Spiegel gave a live demonstration designed to show how easily such false memories can be implanted. In front of colleagues and cameras, he hypnotized a man and told him that communists intended to take over radio and television stations. He gave no details but did suggest to the man that he would remember specific information later. When the session ended, the subject began to talk about the plot, providing an elaborate story complete with details such as a description of the furnishings in the room where he first heard about the planned takeover. He also accepted and incorporated further suggestions given to him by others he talked to, even though no longer in hypnosis. Subsequently rehypnotized, the suggestions were 'removed'. Later, when shown the videotape of the event, he reacted with shock and surprise.

Twelve years later, Spiegel wrote about the episode:

> During the experiment, in response to the hypnotic signal, the subject created a totally false story to rationalize his compliance. He sincerely believed it to be true. Since he was locked into the hypnotic bind, he suspended his own critical judgement. He lied but did not actually know he was lying. At the time, he was in effect *an honest liar.*[24]

Despite Spiegel's classic demonstration, hundreds of subsequent experiments showing a similar effect even without hypnosis, and a growing number of recanters making public statements that their memories uncovered in therapy are false, the Psychology Industry continues to create 'honest liars'. Psychologists continue to use these memories in therapy regardless of their dubious accuracy. Fiore, in her book on past-life therapy, writes: 'whether the former lifetimes that are "lived" are fantasies or actual experiences lived in a bygone era does not matter to me as a therapist – getting results is important.'[25] Another psychologist, with a more traditional approach to psychotherapy, states: 'the retrieval of true, distorted or false memories of abuse can lead to an individual's improvement in therapy. A patient might need to have his/her memories *validated* for therapeutic gains even if these memories are "false," but as long as no harmful steps ensue.'[26] Apparently the Psychology Industry sees no harm in lying to patients, despite the harm that can come from making false accusations based on these memories or from being exposed as liars.

Psychologists involved in memory work hold the belief that what they are doing is for the good of their patient, even if 'the work' involves the patient 'reliving' terrifying experiences akin to horror movies. For instance, a young woman, hospitalized because of continued haemorrhaging after a miscarriage, became upset and asked to be seen by a psychiatrist. When he arrived, she explained that she had been moved into the hospital ward where her mother had died and, fearing that she might be dying too, she had panicked. She was moved to another ward, felt better but still seemed distressed; so he encouraged her to tell him more about what was troubling her. She talked about a bad dream she had had a week before: 'I dreamed that I had an itchy place on my hand . . . And when I scratched it, all these bugs came out of where I was scratching it! Little spiders, just pouring out of the skin on my hand.' The psychiatrist interpreted the dream as 'blatantly symbolic' and suggested the need to 'find out what the dream is revealing from the inside'.

The woman did not want to explore the dream; so, over many sessions, he listened and encouraged her to talk. 'Let it come, as much as you can. Don't judge it, if you can help it. Just let yourself go.' Screaming in terror, the woman began to 'relive memories'. 'It's . . . it's . . . it's all black,' she began. Eventually she described how at the age of five she had been tortured for months in satanic rituals, in which her mother had taken part. She described being forced to watch cult members nail babies to crosses, stab a dead baby with a crucifix, and eat the ashes of a dead woman. After months of such experiences, the little girl lay 'all a mess, her stomach swollen with malnutrition, her flesh flaccid, her eyes vacant, with blood all over. Then, Satan himself appeared.' As these 'images' kept coming, the woman asked whether she might not be making all this up. Her psychiatrist reassured her that he believed her. 'After eight months of therapy, aside from his reassurance, the only 'proof' she had of her ordeal were body memories,' such as 'whenever she relived the moments when Satan had his burning tail wrapped around her neck, a sharply defined rash appeared in the shape of the spade-like tip of his tail.'[27]

It is not only adults who become caught up in reliving such memories. Children are also being encouraged to talk about such bizarre things as if they were real. Entire communities have become caught up in seemingly benevolent efforts to protect these children.

In a quiet North Carolina town, charges of sexual abuse were laid against the owners of a local day-care centre. This followed a conference at which law-enforcement and social-service workers were briefed on the dangers of child molesters in day-care centres. As rumours spread, new meaning was read into children's bruises, tantrums, fears and stories. At least seventy children, most between the ages of three and five, were sent to four state-recommended therapists. Court records show that one of the psychologists, who was the head of the counselling group that had sponsored the conference, had shown a five-year-old girl drawings of satanic symbols, which included a horned mask and inverted crosses, in an effort to uncover instances of devil worship. According to her notes, when the child looked at the mask, she claimed that the day-care owner had worn 'one of those'. Initially having reported only a spanking by this man, after biweekly sessions for six months, the girl was remembering 'oral penetration by a penis, vaginal penetration by a brown felt-tipped marker and witnessing the murder of human babies'. In addressing the delay in getting to this material, the psychologist explained that children can be terrified into silence.[28]

Unfortunately, what people come to believe through revising existing memories or uncovering new ones can lead to dramatic changes in the way they relate to others in their lives. And too often they lead to accusations which have devastating effects.

'You are under arrest and you are charged with sexual assault, rape, gross indecency and uttering a death threat.'

Thus began a man's year-long ordeal, as his car was surrounded by police cars on a public street, while video cameras rolled. For Harold Levy, this day in May 1993 was the beginning, but in fact the events leading up to it went back several years and show what can and does happen to innocent people caught up in the results of memory work.

A young woman known to Levy and his family had entered into treatment for an eating disorder. The psychologist quickly attributed the problem to 'sexual abuse' and referred her to social workers who specialized in this area. One thing led to the other, resulting in 'a chain of horrors', as Levy describes it. Once she was persuaded of the allegations, the police became involved. Without further investigation beyond that of the statement of the accuser, supported by the therapists, they laid charges.

Levy, a prominent lawyer, journalist and law professor, had no idea that anything was going on; he remained completely unaware of any allegations until 'this day in May'. After that, his home was searched and police reported finding pornographic tapes. Ironically, the videotapes were of television shows about accused people whose cases had raised questions about prosecutions; material for a book Levy was writing on the miscarriage of justice.

Almost a year later, the woman recanted the allegations that Levy had sexually assaulted her over many years using knives and beer bottles. Facing the pending trial and finally seeing the gravity of the situation, she had received independent psychological counsel and come to realize how she had been influenced. The charges were dropped.

In a subsequent interview, Levy spoke of the effect on himself and his family. 'You know how they talk of a nuclear family, well, it was like the bomb exploded.' When asked to speculate on what gives psychologists such power to change this woman's mind so that she would come out with both these bizarre allegations and this false image of a man whom she had known for years, he replied:

> I think it's a mixture of several things. They deal with people who are very vulnerable and weak and in crisis and they give them something to latch on to. And these people know how to hand out the victim roles and all the things that go with them: the compassion, the simple explanation of what's wrong with them, what ails them, what troubles them and takes away their peace of mind. They provide them support; they have networks and safe houses. They don't want them to talk to people who might be able to help. They isolate their clients from them. So they have a whole structure of control and influence. And for some reason the public has been hooked in to this and judges listen to them and accept their tyranny because, if you don't go along with them, you are branded.[29]

Levy's lawyer Alan Gold, a prominent defence attorney in Canada, places the responsibility for synthetic victims squarely on the shoulders of psychologists and their professional organizations. In an interview he described how a belief system had grown up over the past decade and become an ideology in which scepticism was not tolerated. Initially, in the mid-eighties, no one questioned the allegations, as psychologists assured the public that they were true: 'no one would lie about something like that.' Once an uncritical foundation was set, not only did unwitting clients come under the influence of these psychologists but so too did the courts and politicians. According to Gold, 'the same psychologist that testifies in court today, conducted the seminar that taught the police how to investigate the case last weekend.' Identifying it as a 'self-contained belief system', he described how police, prosecutors, patients, and the public had all been brought under the influence of these 'purveyors of quackery' who 'want to cripple the whole adult population'. Gold pointed the finger of responsibility directly at the psychology organizations which for years had turned a blind eye to these practices, refusing to challenge their members with the scientific data which contradicted their claims. In many ways, psychologists had a free hand to 'pour into their suggestible clients' whatever belief they wanted, whether it was UFO abduction, past lives or sexual abuse. 'Nobody stood up for the truth' until the early nineties 'when some top scientists began to speak out on their own, independent of their professional organizations which continued their conspiracy of silence'.[30]

False Naming

> *The traumatized person is often relieved simply to learn the true name of her condition. By ascertaining her diagnosis, she begins the process of recovery.*[31]

Traditionally, in medicine, diagnosing or naming a condition has been a source of hope for many patients. The label implies that the physician knows what is wrong, what to do and what the outcome is likely to be. For example, a severe pain in the lower right quadrant of the body, along with an elevated temperature, indicates appendicitis, which suggests that surgery will bring about a good recovery.

However, naming or diagnosing 'diseases' in the pseudo-medical field of the Psychology Industry is mostly fictional in nature. While some forms of mental illness have sufficient physiological factors to be consistently identified (e.g. Alzheimer's and Parkinson's diseases), most of the disorders treated by the Psychology Industry are merely social terms reflecting cultural influences and moral positions. What is considered a psychological illness in one culture or at one time in history, may be seen in another culture as appropriate, eccentric, criminal or spiritual. A case of multiple personality might be seen as a psychological illness, a weird aspect of a nonconforming person or a spirit possession; just as excessive alcohol consumption might be viewed as an addiction, a cultural trait, a quality of the flamboyant artistic personality or a criminal act.

Frank and Frank have identified the moral, the theoretical and the entrepreneurial as three factors which affect this 'naming'.[32] It has been argued that the diagnoses of the Psychology Industry, which are revised frequently, are actually culturally influenced moral judgements which convert the person's behaviour into pathology and make the psychologist an enforcer (or reinforcer) of changing societal values.[33] For instance, the Psychology Industry may pejoratively describe the construction worker who whistles at a passing woman as harassing and assaultive, while being more forgiving of such behaviours as consuming alcohol, using heroin or overeating, calling these 'addictive diseases'.

A diagnosis may just as easily be the product of a theory; for 'variants of normal behaviour and ordinary unhappiness become illnesses amenable to psychotherapy when a theory exists to explain them as such'.[34] Homosexuality was once a diagnosis because psychoanalytic theory offered a pathological explanation for the behaviour, and now high levels of heterosexual activity have become 'sexual addictions', a new theoretical diagnosis which gained prominence with the Clinton affair. As Schofield stated thirty years ago: 'Case finding tends frequently to result in case making . . .' While he argued that 'the individual who is dissatisfied with his work, unhappy in his social relationships, lacking in recreational skills . . . is not helped by sensitization to the notion that he is "sick",'[35] the fabricated victim of today is told that he can benefit from such a label.

The entrepreneurial factor also plays a dramatic role in current diagnostics. Just as 'therapeutic schools unwittingly foster the phenomena which they cure',[36] so too do treatment centres foster the frequency of diagnosis of the problems they treat. For example, profit-oriented residential treatment centres for addictions increased by 350 per cent and their caseloads by 400 per cent between 1978 and 1984.[37]

Whatever underlies the diagnosis, be it social control, theoretical musing or economic greed, 'naming' serves a purpose. While it may give comfort and hope through the implied understanding on the part of the psychologist, it also provides a new identity for the client: 'I am a victim.' Unlike medicine, where an incorrect diagnosis can result in death, no such embarrassing risk exists for the Psychology

Industry; those who get worse or even commit suicide can in retrospect be seen as 'untreatable', while most just languish in their victim status. Meanwhile, as these synthetic victims remain in treatment, not yet recovered, psychologists continue to make their money.

The Psychology Industry relies on the *Diagnostic and Statistical Manual* (the *DSM-IV*) of the American Psychiatric Association, for many of the names and labels it uses.[38] The original 1954 version served to crystallize the nineteenth-century belief that mental illnesses were biologically based and similar to physical diseases. But unlike medical diagnoses that convey a probable cause, appropriate treatment and likely prognosis, the disorders listed in the *DSM-IV* are terms arrived at through peer consensus, designed to be used in communicating information, conducting research, providing treatment and *doing billing.* As Showalter points out in her 1997 book *Hystories: Hysterical Epidemics and Modern Media*, a useful label or diagnosis requires 'at least three ingredients: physician enthusiasts and theorists; unhappy, vulnerable patients; and supportive cultural environments. A doctor or other authority figure must first define, name, and publicize the disorder and then attract patients into its community.'[39]

The brief history of post-traumatic stress disorder (PTSD), one of the Psychology Industry's favourite terms, illustrates this process of evolving labels. PTSD initially appeared in the *DSM* in 1980, legitimizing 'the relentless suffering of Vietnam veterans' and lifting it 'out of the realm of psychopathology into the realm of *fundable* war casualty'. It quickly became a buzzword going far beyond its original patient population, 'bringing added support to thousands of rape victims seeking respect and protection within the legal system'.[40] In the hands of the Psychology Industry, it led to the battlefield being seen as 'a microcosm of trauma',[41] resulting in virtually any scene from everyday life having the potential to be seen as a battlefield. With PTSD as a diagnostic starting point, women could be labeled as 'the casualties of the war of the sexes';[42] verbal insults could be equated with bullets and hurt feelings could be seen as wounds.

Twisting the term, using any tragic or disturbing event as a cause, the Psychology Industry could justify judging people's lives.

In London, a head teacher was stabbed to death when he went to the rescue of a thirteen-year-old student being attacked by a teenage gang. The next day, Cardinal Basil Hume prayed with the 440 children and staff for both the man and his killer. After suggesting how they should be inspired by the headmaster's noble act and reminding them that he was a friend of the pupils and that they were his friends, he said: 'It is right that we should cry. We have to mourn, we have to grieve. It's part of human living. I believe every teacher in this school would have done what Philip Lawrence did.' He urged the killer to contact the police, saying that the young man 'who did this terrible crime has to acknowledge it, he has to be punished for it, he has to pay his debt' and 'we have to try hard in our hearts to forgive.'[43]

While the cardinal focused on the murdered man as a victim, a good person and a friend, a leading psychiatrist was identifying the students as the victims of trauma. Professor Isaac Marks declared them to be at risk of PTSD and recommended immediate counselling. He warned that the children who had seen the attack or held the dying man in their arms 'would suffer a range of feelings varying from detachment to disbelief, mood swings, flashbacks and nightmares'. He suggested that 'some may develop hyper-vigilance, where sufferers constantly worry about their safety', and stated that 'in the coming days and weeks, many youngsters would feel a sense of guilt or responsibility'. He predicted that 'the few who carry the effects for years may find they under-perform at school, or become over-protective towards their loved ones in adulthood.'[44] Using *DSM* terminology, he ignored a real victim and turned a group of mourning friends into a pool of potential synthetic victims.

False naming sometimes involves 'diagnosing' people who have experienced such a tragedy, but often it involves turning confused or unhappy people into victims of one sort or another. For example, a freelance photographer whose wife had left him wondered why and, frustrated by his failed attempts to have another relationship, he saw a psychologist, who diagnosed him as a 'love and sex addict', dependent on love and sex, 'just like alcoholics need alcohol'. Based on this, the psychologist explained how he was experiencing 'withdrawal effects' and prescribed long-term therapy to help him 'uncover the early childhood events which caused him to confuse love and sex and "crave" affection'. He was also referred to a 'love and sex addicts anonymous' group based on the twelve-step approach of AA. In the group, he broke the rules and developed a friendship with one of the women. But when their friendship eventually became amorous, he and the woman felt so guilty that they stopped seeing each other. Because he believed the diagnosis, at no time did this man consider what he might be doing to turn women off, consider the reasons for his wife's infidelity, or feel free to discover what might be good in the new relationship. Since he was labelled an addict, all relationships involving sex, including this latter one, were interpreted as expressions of his addiction. He was caught in a psychological catch-22.

Contrived Victims

Everyone who is born holds dual citizenship, in the kingdom of the well and in the kingdom of the sick.

Susan Sontag

Just as much a product of the Psychology Industry as the synthetic victims are the many seriously ill people persuaded to turn to psychologists for help. Though it is not immediately apparent, their approach involves reshaping their understanding of the medical diagnosis so as to make it appear that, in one way or another, their condition is the result of psychological factors and their survival depends on identifying and controlling these hidden causes. Well-publicized beliefs, along with a long-standing tendency to view ill people as victims, makes it relatively easy for the Psychology Industry to convert them successfully.

Continuous reference to people with heart disease, cancer, AIDS and so on as victims has caused society to become accustomed to thinking about them as unfortunate victims involved in a losing war going on within their own bodies. For centuries people believed that such conditions were the result of humour, phlegm and bile which needed to be drawn out of the body.

However, in the 1950s, the work of Selye and others drew attention to the idea that other factors, particularly psychological and social, can affect health, sparking a resurgence of interest in psychosomatic medicine. From this has emerged the impression that the age-old mystery of the mind–body connection has been solved and invites people to take refuge 'in a fairyland populated with such fuzzy concepts as "stress"'.[45] The Psychology Industry enthusiastically endorses the notion that psychological factors such as stress, anger and depression, whether they be linked to a type of relationship, an event or a lifestyle, make people vulnerable to disease and can be avoided or reversed. For example:

> Stress has been called the silent killer, attacking those who had no previous warning . . . I tell my patients to imagine stress as a heavy knapsack that has some of its compartments filled with sand . . . Our program will help you find the compartments with sand, dump them, and go on your way with a much lighter load.[46]

> Anger kills. We're speaking here not about the anger that drives people to shoot, stab, or otherwise wreak havoc on their fellow humans. We mean instead the everyday sort of anger, annoyance, and irritation that courses through the minds and bodies of many perfectly normal people.[47]

In response to these notions, millions of dollars are spent each year. Pop psychology books rise to the top of the charts, purporting to reveal how to reduce stress and to prevent or treat illnesses ranging from ulcers to heart attacks and cancer, from asthma to allergies and AIDS.[48] The Psychology Industry makes claims about how laughter works as a remedy, how curbing anger can save your life, how optimism cures. Pretending to have discovered the psychological equivalent of penicillin but unable to demonstrate comparable shifts in disease and death rates, it continues to applaud itself for its essential contribution to health care.

It claims that between '40 to 60% of visits to physicians stem from psychological problems' and that 'psychologists are extremely well-suited to contribute to the care of these patients.'[49] It employs the image of the psychologist as 'doctor', 'healer', 'compassionate listener', along with the language of science, to achieve its objective. It convinces patients that psychological factors played a role in their getting sick and that conversely they can, with the help of the Psychology Industry, 'control their stress', 'enhance their positive emotions', 'boost their immunity', 'fight their cancer cells' and 'get well again'. Instead of being medical patients with a biological disease, they are manufactured into contrived victims of a psychological disorder.

The best-known and most effective money-makers in this system have been the relaxation procedures to deal with cardiovascular diseases and the 'mind–body' techniques for fighting immune disorders such as cancer and AIDS.

Early studies suggested that individuals who were aggressive, competitive, work-oriented and with a constant sense of urgency had a greater risk of a heart attack, and that they needed to change and develop a 'relaxation response'. However, the many programmes that have been developed and marketed to change personality patterns or to teach relaxation skills have proven to be of little clinical value.[50]

Also popular, and probably of greater overall commercial effect, have been the plethora of the 'mind–body' programmes offered to help terminally ill people 'fight' their disease. In the mid-1970s, Carl and Stephanie Simonton attracted public attention with their book *Getting Well Again*,[51] in which they presented a psychological programme described as 'an important weapon in the "war on cancer"'. People who might have been emotionally strong and capable throughout most of their lives and were now diagnosed with cancer were being told that they were:

- Not as strong as they thought.
- Succumbing to the stresses in their lives.
- Partially to blame for the cancer.
- Needing help to deal with their emotions.[52]

Although the treatment programmes for these contrived victims claim to be 'well supported by scientific data', they have failed to deliver the promised cures. Today their proponents are likely to hedge their bets with such statements as 'even if the disease cannot be slowed down, living life in a fulfilling fashion, feeling good about yourself, and leaving your body in a peaceful way are worthwhile goals . . .'

While it would be absurd to deny a connection between the mind and the body or to refuse seriously ill people the compassion they deserve, there is no basis on which to assume that the Psychology Industry holds the key to the mystery or the monopoly on caring.

Counterfeit Victims

Lest men suspect your tale to be untrue,
Keep probability – some say – in view . . .
Sigh then, or frown, but leave (as in despair)
Motive and end and moral, in the air;
Nice contradiction between fact and fact
Will make the whole read human and exact.

Robert Graves

He 'put the screwdriver in my vagina, the handle, and then he put the other one in my rectum' and then he 'moved both the screwdrivers at the same time while they were inside of me.' He said 'Just lay there like a good little girl,' as he 'took the screwdrivers out of my vagina and rectum' and eventually 'pushed his penis into my vagina . . .'[53]

This statement to the police launched a manhunt for a violent rapist who had abducted the woman at gunpoint and taken her to an underground garage where he raped and sodomized her. The woman was referred to a 'women's sexual assault centre' where she received counselling. A door-to-door campaign was launched to alert the public and a search was begun. In a subsequent statement, the young woman described the assault taking place in a dark park area, and later she disclosed that she had the name and address of the man.

When arrested, the shocked young man said that he had met the woman at a bar and had invited her back to his apartment where they had consensual sex. He reported that they were not alone in the house and that, in fact, when his landlady had intruded on them at one point, the young woman had made no effort to protest or seek help. She had been fully willing. He had even given his name and address to her, hopeful that they might meet again. After his arrest and statement, the woman changed her story.

With this and other information gathered by the police, it became clear that no attack had taken place. The police charged the woman with public mischief, to which she responded: 'How can you charge me, you can't prove I consented to the sex.'

Meanwhile, she continued to receive counselling from a social worker and a psychiatrist at a sexual-assault centre. At the trial, the psychiatrist testified that, regardless of the facts, the woman was suffering from post-traumatic stress disorder owing to the trauma of rape. She claimed that it is typical in these cases that the women are confused and unable to remember the events clearly, a result of what she called 'rape trauma syndrome'. She interpreted the event the woman had reported to the police as an instance of 'date rape'.

The psychiatrist also claimed that the woman had actually been raped before, when she was twelve years old, and was now confusing that event with the more recent one. Although there was no corroboration of the claim of an earlier assault and the woman could not even recall it, the psychiatrist went on record saying: 'give me ten years with this woman and I will help her remember that she was raped.'

Despite the lies and attempts to mislead the police, the arrest of an innocent man, and the parroting of 'explanations, words and ideas given to her by others', the judge acquitted the woman, concluding that she was 'suffering from some sort of stress disorder'.

Why would she make up such a story? There are several possible motives. She had a somewhat uninterested boyfriend. Perhaps the rape story was intended to rekindle this passion, or maybe she needed an alibi for coming in late that evening or just an excuse for having had a sexual encounter that she wished, on reflection, had not occurred.

Counterfeit victims often invent their stories, as this woman did, 'in the heat of the moment' or as a way to cope with some pressure or situation. The Psychology Industry provides the themes, the encouragement, the support and, often, the validation. Assault, rape and harassment, being highly publicized and emotionally charged issues, are some of the more popular themes. In some circles, it is considered improper to question the truthfulness of a story. But psychologically inspired fictional tales are often told. One study conducted in a small metropolitan area in the Midwestern United States looked at the excuses given by women who, having taken their stories to the police, later admitted that no rape had occurred.[54] The reasons given generally fell into three categories:

(1) creating an alibi,
(2) seeking revenge following rejection or disappointment,
(3) wanting attention or sympathy.

The model of the counterfeit victim is neither complicated nor foreign. Like the child saying 'he made me do it', it is something that is familiar to everyone. It begins with being in a jam, needing an excuse, wanting attention or affection, or venting anger and seeking revenge.

The comedienne Roseanne Barr, whose volatile relationship with her husband Tom Arnold became as public as their television shows, presented herself for a time as a battered wife, describing how Arnold had 'pushed, pummelled and pinched her'. But four days after making up with him and dropping divorce proceedings, she withdrew the charges, saying: 'I signed an uncorrected, unread copy of a letter from my divorce lawyer in anger and haste . . . He never beat me. He never abused me. Although it's a titillating story to many out there, it is untrue and insults women who really are battered.'[55]

Barr's allegations of abuse, which some suspected were born out of a desire for revenge, disappeared as quickly as they had surfaced. But not all counterfeit victims find it so easy to shrug off the lies. Katie Roiphe describes how Mindy, a student at Princeton who had fabricated a rape story, was forced publicly to admit her lie.

> She claimed she had reported a rape, and she hadn't . . . She told people that a certain male undergraduate was the rapist, and he complained to the administration. Mindy responded to administrative pressure by printing an apology in the student newspaper, explaining the motivation as political: 'I made my statements in the *Daily Princeton* and at the Take Back the Night March in order to raise awareness for the plight of the campus rape victims' and describing how she had 'in several personal conversations and especially at the Take Back the Night March, [been] overcome by emotion . . .'[56]

Although these cases and thousands like them gain little public notice, they affect tens of thousands of people who are misled or falsely accused. Sometimes the accused are cleared, though many, in the interim, incur huge legal costs and suffer damage to their families and their reputations, and sometimes they are convicted and forced to serve sentences for acts they never committed. The allegations are usually supported by the Psychology Industry. Rape trauma, battered-wife syndrome, abuse, incest – a whole range of possibilities exist for people to tailor to their own particular needs.

And since the majority of the Psychology Industry's consumers, and most accusers, are women, the options are packaged to appear anti-patriarchal and pro-feminist. They are presented in popular magazines, TV talk shows, movies and sitcoms. Roseanne Barr may have picked up the idea for her accusation, as she claimed, from her lawyer, or possibly she read it in a script for one of her own shows. Whatever her source, women are constantly being presented with such ideas.

The *Ladies' Home Journal*, in an article on 'Stress Sex', tells women: 'We all know that stress can make us do crazy things. Now, according to a ground-breaking theory, it may be the reason more and more wives are cheating on their husbands. How stressed-out – and vulnerable to infidelity – are *you*?' It continues: 'as many as 55% of wives cheat on their husbands,' and it describes what used to be called 'adultery' or simply 'having an affair' as 'stress-induced-straying'. No longer can a woman participate and even enjoy succumbing to passion, seducing a man or being seduced.

> Although a woman who's stressed may well be aware of just how tired or angry she is, or how little the reality of her life matches what she thought it would be, she may *not* be conscious of how much she longs for the recreation, emotional connection and sexual passion she no longer enjoys. But below the surface, the longing is there, and it makes her uniquely vulnerable to an extramarital fling.[57]

No longer does she need to entertain responsibility or guilt for an affair; she can claim that stress made her do it.

These psychological excuses can be extended beyond the relatively trivial misbehaviour of an extramarital fling all the way to murder. Psychologists who have studied women who kill their children, report that 'severe depression or an unbearable "pileup of stresses" may trigger latent emotional or mental illness'.[58] A University of New Hampshire psychologist states that those who kill are 'sometimes women who have very low self-esteem, or women who feel that they have the possibility of a relationship and the man doesn't want the responsibility of kids'.[59]

While women are the more common users of such excuses, the

most famous counterfeit victim in the history of American justice remains a man known as 'the Hillside Strangler'. Kenneth Bianchi abducted and strangled ten young women in Los Angeles before being arrested in Washington for two additional murders. A total of eight psychologists became involved at various stages of the case.[60]

Bianchi, who had studied psychology and impersonated a psychologist in a counselling practice, was better prepared than most to be a counterfeit victim. When arrested, the evidence against him was strong; he was likely to be convicted and executed. Claiming that he could remember nothing about the night of 11 January beyond having gone for a drive, he began to draw psychologists, their method and their beliefs, into his defence. The first psychologist hinted to Bianchi that multiple personality disorder (MPD) might be the explanation for his amnesia. Another recommended hypnosis as a means to uncover the repressed memories. A third concluded that the amnesia was an indicator of MPD. Eventually a psychiatrist, Martin Orne, hired by the prosecution, demonstrated that Bianchi was faking hypnosis and argued convincingly that Bianchi was conning 'the experts'.[61]

Cases such as Bianchi's, while they receive media attention, do not portray the typical counterfeit victim. It is rather the countless other liars who are never exposed or whose lies have become so commonplace that they are merely shrugged off, who serve the industry much better. These are the more common pretenders, who fabricate stories and feign symptoms based on themes provided by the Psychology Industry.

Medicine has long been aware of a small proportion of patients who pretend to be suffering from a particular physical illness for no apparent reason other than attention.[62] In its most extreme form, Munchausen syndrome, individuals consent to undergo extremely painful tests and major surgery, and may even bleed, poison and mutilate themselves in order to appear sick. Until recently the faking of psychological symptoms has been considered even more rare than the feigning of physical symptoms. But the growth of the victim-making industry, with the proliferation of information about psychological conditions and the growth of services to cater to them, may be leading to an epidemic, not of MPD or violence, but rather of 'playing sick'. Some people fake symptoms and make up stories because they want to belong to a group, receive attention and gain support. But such individuals are only one segment of a much larger group of counterfeit victims who take on a wide variety of roles, for reasons ranging from getting their way at work, at home or in court, to defrauding insurance companies or establishing alibis for murder.

One of the jurors in the O. J. Simpson trial was released from duty because she had earlier reported to the police that she had been a victim of domestic violence. Subsequently, Jeanette Harris admitted that the accusations of battering and marital rape were false, stating: 'I have never ever been a victim of domestic abuse.' When asked why she had made the claims when she knew them to be untrue, she replied: 'It was just a part of a custody dispute; nobody believed that.'

But such accusations are not benign. Legal experts estimate that up to 20 per cent of custody disputes are complicated by unsupported reports of abuse. So serious is the situation that a 1998 Canadian Joint Committee of the Senate and Parliament, investigating issues of custody and access, considered the option of criminalizing such false accusations.[63]

A similar problem exists with claims of sexual harassment. While the official statement of the APA, unsupported by any credible data, has read that 'research shows that less than one percent of complaints are false',[64] lawyers specializing in this area offer very different numbers with a much broader range and generally much higher. One US lawyer suspects that upwards of 15 per cent of claims are made by counterfeit victims and 60–70 per cent by synthetic victims.[65]

While physical injuries have, for a long time, been a common basis for insurance claims and civil law suits, the victim-making capacity of the Psychology Industry has facilitated a rapidly growing business of financial claims based on psychological injuries. Like the 'soft-tissue damage' claims, some real and some feigned, which can never be seen on X-rays or lab tests, psychological damages are invisible. When accompanied by the supportive report of a psychologist and a confirming diagnosis, insurance payoffs can range from time off work to a compensation package, and civil lawsuits can yield payments for specific damages (the trouble sleeping, the nightmares, the fatigue), general damages (the loss of 'enjoyment of life' or 'ability to enjoy sex') and punitive damages.

All of this has become so routine that virtually no one questions the role psychologists are playing in these scams; often insurance claims are simply processed and lawsuits are settled out of court. Whereas psychologists at one time were expected to investigate injury claims and to make an effort to detect malingerers, even to the point of challenging people on their motives, the Psychology Industry today, when it comes to assessing psychological damages, tends toward a nod of approval. What the patient says, whether based on fact or revenge, financial gain or some other motive, and often regardless of conflicting information, is accepted as true. Whether it is out of naivety, fear of reprimand[66] or basic self-interest, psychologists seem disinclined or dumb to the notion of questioning the client and, on occasion, uncovering the counterfeit victim.

In talking about the various forms of therapy that exist, Kottler concluded that the overall goal of psychological treatment is 'satisfied clients'.[67] It would seem, with regard to counterfeit victims, that the Psychology Industry is so dedicated to this principle of customer satisfaction that it welcomes liars, encourages lying and provides endless opportunities for the support of all victims, including the counterfeits.

The Cost of Fabricated Victimhood

And this is the way the world will end
Not with a bang, but a whimper.

T. S. Eliot

In pursuit of its 'satisfied customers', the Psychology Industry ignores its ethical and professional responsibility to consider the long-term effects of its activities on individuals and on society.

First and foremost is the harm being done to authentic victims. When so many 'cry victim', it becomes almost impossible to know what is true and what is false. As Charles Sykes has pointed out, 'When everyone is a victim, then no one is.'[68]

While the Psychology Industry incessantly promotes its efforts to decrease violence in society, and to protect and help victims, its primary effect is to divert attention and resources into its own concepts of violence and into its own bogus solutions. It has encouraged whining and blaming to the point where the demands of its users are drowning out the cries of real victims. When one examines the actual effects of the industry's efforts on the victims of brutal crimes, wars and local tragedies, one finds these individuals often mythologized, ignored or left to their own fate. Through influencing the legal system to be sensitive to 'subtle cues' of abuse, intolerant of relatively trivial acts, and validating the accusations, excuses and claims of both honest and intentional liars, it is fostering a backlash against authentic victims. The search for 'truth' amid the psychologizing, pathologizing and generalizing of the Psychology Industry is wreaking such havoc on American society that 'crying victim' (even if the assault or rape, abuse or battering is for real) may soon inspire dispassion and disbelief.

Fabricated victims of all types run the risk of becoming trapped and tangled up in their victim identities. Unsure of their ability to take care of themselves, they become dependent, immature and helpless, needing protection, support and 'nurturance'. Surrendering their autonomy, self-determination and personal power, they come to be identified as helpless individuals, lacking the ability to think clearly and make decisions. 'Protected' from situations that test or demand their abilities to deal with conflict, they resign themselves to the unreal compassion and soothing of therapeutic, self-help and support-group relationships. Cutting themselves off from family members and friends who may challenge and confront their beliefs, they lose their roots both in their personal histories and in their communities. Tied only to psychologists, who remain 'allies' only as long as funds last, they enter a 'freefall' into eventual self-destruction.

The counterfeit victims, even those whose initial lie may have been said in the heat of the moment, find that with each modification, elaboration or 'validation' of their story, it becomes more and more difficult to take back the lie, which may become the central, enduring theme of their lives. Synthetic victims too can become trapped, as they become accustomed to feeling, appearing, sounding and behaving like victims, incorporating whatever suggestions are offered by the Psychology Industry into their new understanding of themselves and their lives. For the contrived victims, their acceptance of Psychology Industry explanations and proffered hope can often mean that they waste precious time and resources on false explanations and unfounded hopes.

Moreover, fabricated victims, especially those who accuse others of crimes and evil acts, run the increasing risk of eventually experiencing guilt and shame, and possible humiliation and blame. Counterfeits can be exposed, and run the increasing risk of public humiliation and criminal prosecution. And to some extent, synthetic victims run the same risk. Their lies too can be exposed and, as society becomes more aware of these deceptions, it will become both less believing and less tolerant of all fabricated victims. At some point, it will quit trying to tell the difference between the 'honest' and the intentional liar, and judge all of them the same, demanding 'the truth' and punishing the liars. It is conceivable, too, that those falsely and unfairly accused will stop thinking kindly of naive synthetic victims, and that even 'recanters' will find themselves unable to hold psychologists responsible for the actions they have taken based on false interpretations and memories.

The Psychology Industry is separating people from their families, promoting stereotypic and hostile views of men and women, degrading friendship, and generally promoting distrust and suspicion. While no one would condone serious abuse, the Psychology Industry re-interprets vague recollections, making minor events sinister. And while no one would excuse domestic violence, the

Psychology Industry blurs the concept and ignores the context. The Psychology Industry promotes fear and inequality, treating all interpersonal relationships as potentially threatening. It is teaching people to see others as potential enemies, to be monitored, scrutinized and accused. As a result, it is squelching the human tendencies to trust, to flirt, to seduce, to argue and yell, to assume responsibility, to be cautious, to take risks, to be passionate, to make the right choices and to make mistakes. It has created a sense of distance between people and a sense that the only ones to be trusted are the psychologists.

3

Selling Psychology as Science

There are in fact two things, science and opinion; the former begets knowledge, the latter ignorance.

Hippocrates

Society is easily convinced of the value of anything characterized as science. In a gullible way, people believe that a product is better if described as 'proven effective' or 'scientifically developed', whether it is a toothpaste, a new drug, a government 'study' or a therapy.

Whatever the product being promoted, the term 'science' is there to influence the consumer. Advertisers have found that consumers will believe that something is good if it is called 'scientific', even if science has become confused with surveys, opinion polls, celebrity endorsements, advertising slogans and journalistic hype.

So it is hardly surprising that 'science' has become the Gucci label of the Psychology Industry, enhancing its credibility by implying quality, reliability and excellence. But are the 'facts' given by the Psychology Industry based on science? Can they be relied on when making decisions or creating policies? Are the services and treatments of the Psychology Industry safe? Are they effective? Is psychology a science? Or is it just using 'science' to sell itself?

In addressing these questions, one must ask whether the studies it refers to are genuinely scientific, whether the terms and concepts it uses are valid, and whether the data it produces and cites are reliable.

And one must look at whether the Psychology Industry subjects its products to scientific evaluation and how it responds to the research findings.

One hundred years ago, William James wrote, 'I wish by treating Psychology like a natural science, to help her become one.'[1] During the first half of the twentieth century, psychology did grow as a science, as evident in the areas of physiological, behavioural and cognitive psychology. The other 'softer' areas, including personality, social, educational and clinical psychology, acquired some aspects of the scientific approach but were greatly influenced by the demands, from within the profession and without, to provide society with immediately useful applications and solutions. This pressure and the associated incentives of prestige and profit worked to the detriment of psychology as a science.

For the most part, psychology, which abandoned philosophy in the 1890s, had, by the 1990s, abandoned science. As a philosophy, it had a soul, a legitimate territory of study and a theoretical style of thinking. As a science, it had a mind, a recognized focus of enquiry and an empirical approach to data. What is now called 'psychology' is, to use Huber's term, 'junk science', swept along by the shifting ground of popular belief and the ephemeral demands for expert opinion. There is little, if any, similarity between this pseudoscience and the real science on which psychology was founded.

Science functions on the principle that for something to be more than subjective opinion or personal belief, it has to be objectively demonstrated. Although the requirement of objectivity is widely accepted by all the mature sciences, the Psychology Industry often fails to take it seriously. The vast majority of psychologists either see no need to support their claims or present fraudulent and misleading 'data'. While they argue that their methods are effective, they rely on 'clinical experience and judgement' or 'case studies' as evidence, effectively ruling out any external verification. As disquieting as this may be, in the Psychology Industry, scientific principles are violated, research is ignored and, in some cases, data are misinterpreted or even fabricated to fit the need.

Faked and Fishy Data

Man's major foe is deep within him. But the enemy is no longer the same. Formerly it was ignorance; today it is falsehood.

Jean-Francois Revel[2]

A major North American breast-cancer study recently concluded that removing a cancerous lump was just as effective as removal of the entire breast; a finding which encouraged many women to have lumpectomies rather than mastectomies.[3] It was subsequently uncovered that at least one contributor to the study, an eminent Montreal physician and university professor, had submitted falsified data.[4]

Such flagrant dishonesty is seldom uncovered in medical research but in psychology it may actually be prevalent. One well known case is that of Sir Cyril Burt, a British school psychologist and eugenicist. By 1943, he had published his first study supporting the claim that intelligence is an inherited trait.[5] In that and subsequent studies, his results strongly supported the 'genetic inheritance' theory and, 'for many years, the central evidence cited to support the claims that IQ is a highly heritable trait was the massive life's work of the late Sir Cyril Burt'.[6]

In the early 1970s, contradictions, ambiguities and absurdities began to be noticed in Burt's writings, raising questions about his data. In 1976 Oliver Gillie, medical correspondent for the London *Sunday Times*, wrote a front-page article exposing Burt as guilty of major scientific fraud. Gillie had attempted to locate Burt's two associates who, according to Burt, had done the IQ testing and co-authored papers with him. Burt's colleagues had never seen them, neither had secretaries, students or other staff at University College. Apparently, neither they nor any of the identical twins that they had supposedly tested had ever existed. A subsequent biography showed that Burt had collected no data at all during the last thirty years of his life, those years in which he published the definitive studies on intelligence.[7]

This would have been merely an embarrassment to Burt's supporters, were it not for the breadth of influence his claims have had. As a result of his convincing arguments, England established the policy that an IQ test be given to all children in their eleventh year, to measure their 'innate intelligence'. The results were used, together with conventional exams, to stream children into separate and unequal school systems. Similar but less rigid approaches were established in both the United States and the Commonwealth. If one accepts that education has an effect on children's futures in terms of employment, earning power and status, then the influence of Burt's fraudulent findings has damaged whole generations.

The sin of both the physician and Sir Cyril Burt was that they provided fake or fishy data which others accepted, and upon which policies were established and decisions made. Although the exposure of such fraud is rare, it is not unusual for statistics to be presented, articles and books to be published, and conclusions to be drawn on the basis of fishy data or in the absence of any supporting evidence.

Abuse of Numbers

> *You know what they say about smoking; it's one of the leading causes of statistics.*
>
> Arthur Black, CBC Radio

As has often been said, 'numbers don't lie', but numbers can help people to lie more convincingly, becoming the basis for statements that are false. For example, in November 1993, media sources throughout North America carried the results of a Canadian government study that found:

> 98 per cent of Canadian women have personally experienced sexual violation,

> 51 per cent of women (sixteen and over) have been the victims of rape or attempted rape, and
> 40 per cent of women reported at least one experience of rape.[8]

The Canadian national news carried the headline: 'Two out of three Canadian women have been sexually assaulted.' Could this be true? Or is this a case of 'data rape'?[9]

The answer lies with the numbers and how they were gathered. While expressing national incidence rates, the results were based on interviews with only 420 women in one Canadian city. The women interviewed were clearly not representative of Canadian women in general. Those over sixty-four years of age were excluded. And 46.5 per cent of the group had a university degree whereas only 7.8 per cent of Canadian women are university graduates.

The sampling itself suggest that this survey was designed with political rather than scientific intentions, as do the data collected. Neil Gilbert refers to this type of data as 'advocacy numbers', intended, as he says,

> to persuade the public that a problem is vastly larger than commonly recognized. Advocacy numbers are derived not through outright deceit but through a more subtle process of distortion. Under the veil of social science, rigorous research methods are employed to measure a problem defined so broadly that it forms a vessel into which almost any human difficulty can be poured.[10]

'Fear' and 'violence' are such broadly defined terms. For instance, this study reported that 56.7 per cent of women experienced 'difficulty sleeping due to fear'. However, the specific question asked was '*Was there ever a time in your life* when you had trouble sleeping, or staying asleep at night, because you were nervous about or afraid for your personal safety?'[11] This question relates to the whole life period of the woman (including childhood). The data shows that for 100 of these women, the fear lasted for 'up to one month' (the shortest category available in the interview). No attempt was made to discern whether any of these women experienced medical problems or other causes of sleep disturbance, which reportedly affect a significant proportion of the adult population.

This serves as merely one example of the misleading nature of the data and conclusions. Despite its violation of scientific principles, organizations no less prestigious than the Canadian Psychological Association have endorsed the report and allowed it to influence the establishment of gender-biased legislation.

While this study serves as an example of the misuse of data to support this strong bias and political cause, it by no means stands alone. One other example is an oft quoted study sponsored by *Ms.* magazine which stated that 25 per cent of all women have been raped by the time they are in college, based on a question which did not ask women whether they had been raped but rather whether they had ever 'given in to sexual intercourse when [they] didn't want to because [they] were overwhelmed by a man's continual arguments and pressure'. Of these women, who were categorized as rape victims, 73 per cent did not define their experience as 'rape'. Mary Kiss, the psychologist conducting the study, defined it as rape, stating that the women themselves didn't recognize what had really happened to them.[12]

Research findings, just because they have lots of numbers, receive government support or are reported in the media, are not necessarily scientific. The Psychology Industry is very effective in misusing its numbers to support current political views and to sell itself.

Abuse of Concepts

Means not, but blunders round about a meaning;
And he whose fustian's so sublimely bad,
It is not poetry, but prose run mad.

Alexander Pope

Whether it is post-traumatic stress disorder (PTSD), used to describe

Vietnam veterans' reactions to napalm attacks, or a woman's reaction to an unwanted whistle, or 'addiction', which can refer to a dependence on heroin or a desire to spend money shopping, terms that previously had meaning are now being abused. The practitioners of pseudoscience have discovered that if they couch their fictions in professional terms, their ideas take on the air of scientific validity and by appropriating someone else's asset of credibility, they can bolster their own.

One example is 'learned helplessness', a well-researched behavioural paradigm, which describes how people affected by one situation can act helpless in another. Learned helplessness was first identified in the animal learning laboratory. In research designed to study avoidance behaviour, dogs were subjected to electric shocks and then observed to see whether they could learn new behaviours to avoid the shock. Seligman and Maier discovered that when there was nothing the dogs could do to stop the shock, they became so passive that later, when avoidance was possible, they failed to act. They had learned to act helpless.

> Learned helplessness in people came to be understood as consisting of three essential characteristics:
> 1) The person gives up and fails to deal with the demands of a situation in which effective coping is possible.
> 2) This follows in the wake of events in which the person had no way to exert any control, as distinct from bad or traumatic events where doing something might have been possible.
> 3) It is due to particular ways of responding that develop during the time of the uncontrollable events and are generalized to new and different situations.

The model of learned helplessness can be used to explain specific psychological problems. For instance, depression may, in some circumstances, be related to a situation in which there is no control. The 'helplessness' is then generalized to other situations so that one reacts in an unnecessarily passive manner; as depressed.

Despite its share of controversy, learned helplessness has maintained credibility within the scientific community. Because it deals with uncontrollable events, passivity and failure, the victim-making industry has often extrapolated and distorted this concept to explain all manner of human problems.

Nicky Marone used the concept in a book portrayed as a 'guide to overcoming learned helplessness'.[13] The author is described as trained in educational psychology, a workshop and seminar leader on learned helplessness, and a consultant to 'numerous organizations, universities and Fortune 500 companies', leading readers to assume that she is an expert in learned helplessness. However, what she writes, as illustrated in Figure 1, bears virtually no relationship to the original behavioural concept established.[14]

In 'selling' the need for treatment, Marone claims that 'Learned Helplessness is a debilitating breakdown in our belief system that can produce serious behaviour disorders. Fortunately this style of behaviour can be unlearned, but, *left untreated, it can ruin a life that would otherwise be happy and fulfilling.*'[15] However, research shows that learned helplessness has a time course, gradually diminishing over a moderate timespan, and not progressing in the absence of treatment. The writer may be right in assuming that many women don't achieve their dreams (as is probably the case with many men), but to attribute this to learned helplessness is to distort the theory, confuse the public, and use science to sell psychotherapy, targeting women as consumers.

PTSD is misused in much the same way. The concept has been stretched and blurred so that 'trauma' has come to be understood as any subjectively disturbing or upsetting event, whether real or imagined. With this highly diluted definition, it can be found in everyone's life and then used to explain subsequent problems. Whether it is hearing others' tragic tales, being criticized in public, or having the delusion of being abducted by a UFO, all are thought to produce PTSD. Common sense could discriminate the difference between the battlefield or a violent rape and a scary television movie or a verbal insult, but psychologists abuse the concept to sell their services.

Concepts such as learned helplessness and PTSD are particularly

FIGURE 1

Criterion	*Marone's Version*	*The Concept of 'Learned Helplessness'*
1) Inappropriate helplessness	'Learned helplessness ensnares a woman in a tangled web of paralysing beliefs, emotions, and behaviours. She consistently doubts herself even when she performs at consistently high levels.'	This notion of performance 'at a high level' conflicts with the aspect of helpless passivity.
2) Previous uncontrollable event	'The study of learned helplessness has unearthed many intriguing insights . . . girls of high ability . . . are the group most debilitated by confusion; that is, they give up.' Later she refers to 'the grim realities of learned helplessness . . . the terrible toll it takes on a woman's life.'	The scientific concept holds that learned helplessness is the result of specific learning experiences in situations in which there is no possibility for control. It is not based on personality or gender.
3) Helpless thinking is generalized	'Learned helplessness corrodes self-esteem, blocks ambition . . . People who suffer from learned helplessness . . . exhibit deficiencies in strategic planning, and are often unable to assess the causes of both their failures and their successes.'	In contrast, the learned-helplessness paradigm considers the generalizing of helpless behaviours and does not confuse itself with issues of self-esteem or ambition and does not accommodate successes.

attractive to the Psychology Industry precisely because they have gained general scientific acceptance. Moreover, since they link psychological problems to uncontrollable situations, they have particular appeal in a society obsessed with personal control. Peterson offers a caution to this sales promotion: 'an over-riding belief in one's own control presents two problems: it brings increased depression in its wake, and it makes meaning in one's life difficult to find.'[16]

False data from nonexistent studies, numbers misinterpreted to support ideologies, terms distorted to expand markets; these are some of the things that the Psychology Industry offers as reputable science. And it is getting away with it for, as Huber notes: 'it is in the healing business that the temptations of junk science are the strongest and the controls against it the weakest.'[17]

Psychotherapy Evaluation

> *Most therapists, I suspect, have been rather traumatized by the research literature: the lack of hard evidence that any form of therapy really 'does any good' in the way that it is supposed to is something to set the seeds of panic sprouting in those who can see no obvious alternative way of making a living.*
>
> David Smail[18]

One would assume, considering the use of psychological services by millions each year, that indisputable evidence exists proving the effectiveness of psychotherapy. But most of the information about therapy's usefulness comes from those who buy and sell the services rather than from scientific research.

Early in the twentieth century, Freud argued against scientific evaluation of psychoanalysis, stating that only the patient could accurately assess its effectiveness, a view that was supported and restated more recently in the *American Handbook of Psychiatry*:

> For the patient, his immediate knowledge of the effect of analysis is sufficient evidence of its worth, however sceptical the outside observer may be and however lacking the statistics to 'prove' its usefulness. Perhaps its effectiveness can never be shown by scientific methods . . . Perhaps the experience of analysis is like that of beauty, of mysticism, of love – self-evident and world-shaking to him who knows it, but quite incommunicable to another who does not.[19]

However, the psychoanalyst Allen Wheelis disputes this, saying: 'few analyzed persons are critical of psychoanalysis.' He notes that if a patient does acknowledge the lack of usefulness, he 'will blame himself and exonerate the psychoanalysis. The most common outcome, however, is simply to pretend that the analysis was successful.' This opinion was inadvertently supported by the Central Fact-Gathering Committee of the American Psychoanalytic Association which reported that of those who 'completed treatment', over 96 per cent 'felt benefitted'.[20]

But the client is not the only one to imagine a cure. Studies consistently show that therapists tend to see more improvement than anyone else, followed closely by their clients. Friends, family and other observers come in a distant, and often unimpressed, third.

Why would psychologists distort the truth, accentuating the positive and minimizing negative results? Of the many reasons, two stand out: looking honestly at what they are doing might interfere with their practice and their income, and might create doubts about their effectiveness, self-worth and chosen career.

Most psychologists offer services in the form of regimented office visits. Regardless of their theoretical orientation, they strive to establish trust, uncover the past, make interpretations or suggestions and develop insight. If research failed to support this approach, the traditional structure could crumble.

People are usually resistant to changing their method of doing business even when confronted with the necessity to do so. Consider the example of Semmelweis who, in the mid-1800s, noted that new mothers served by physicians had almost four times as high a death rate from childbed fever as those assisted by a midwife. He reasoned that the doctors' failure to wash their hands before doing deliveries was the cause. He insisted that his colleagues clean their hands in a solution of chlorine of lime and over a fifteen-month period, the death rate dropped from 12 per cent to 1.2 per cent. Later, his successor stopped the silly and 'unmanly' practice and the death rate rose again to 15 per cent, but this did not persuade the physicians to change their habit until Lister, forty years later, understanding the significance of Semmelweis's reasoning, reinstated hand washing. Despite the importance of Semmelweis's insight, professional practice won out over scientific evidence, in much the same way that the Psychology Industry now maintains traditional practices, ignoring results that cast doubts on their effectiveness.

Psychologists have historically been loath to evaluate their work, preferring to rely on case studies that serve to demonstrate positive outcomes. One admitted: 'Like all therapists, I am constantly looking for signs that the work I'm doing is really helping people.'[21] Like the tall stories told by fishing cronies, these tales of success enhance psychologists' confidence, impress their colleagues and evoke admiration in clients and prospective clients. To admit to failures when colleagues are claiming high success would put a psychologist in jeopardy. It is easier to remember only the successes and blame failure on the patients, calling them 'untreatable', 'too resistant' or just 'not psychologically minded'.

Clients are also prone to exaggerate the effectiveness of their therapy. Zilbergeld points out that the reason 'has to do with the basic nature of counselling: it is, for most people, a very personal, even intimate, matter . . . And the therapist is often supportive, understanding, sympathetic . . . It's hard to say that this kind of relationship or process is useless or harmful, just as it's hard to say that praying is useless even when your prayers aren't answered.'[22]

Rather than being the best suited to evaluate therapy, psychologists and their clients are the least able to answer the questions:

- Is therapy effective?
- Is it any better than friendship?
- Do high-paid professionals do a better job than minimally trained counsellors?
- Does training and experience improve a therapist's skill?
- Is therapy always safe?
- Do professionals know more about human nature than the rest of us?
- Would people naturally get worse without professional treatment?

They say yes to all of these questions while scientific studies that address them are concluding a resounding

NO!

People have the undeniable right to make choices that affect their own lives, whether good or bad. As Morris Parloff, chief of psychotherapy research at the National Institute of Mental Health, says: 'It is an individual's inalienable right to seek therapy, self-enhancement, education, enlightenment, and titillation as long as he or she is willing to pay for it.'[23] But their choice should be made in the clear light of research.

This 'NO' is a warning – an invitation to look more closely at the claims that psychotherapy works.

When something is purported to be 'proven effective', one assumes that it has been carefully tested. Drugs cannot be marketed until they have proven more effective than placebos and of no serious risk to users. Can it be said that psychotherapy is more effective than a placebo and will not harm the patient?

One of the first studies to address this issue was conducted by the British psychologist Hans Eysenck in 1952.[24] In 7,293 psychotherapy cases, he found an improvement rate of 64 per cent, a finding which initially seemed supportive of psychotherapy. However, Eysenck compared these results with those of 500 patients who had received little or no treatment. This 'control group' had made health claims for psychoneurotic disability, had taken at least three months off work due to the problems, but had received no psychotherapy, merely being reassured and given some mild sedatives by their physicians. Eysenck discovered that 72 per cent of them had improved by the second year and that they showed an overall 90 per cent recovery in five years, leading him to conclude that 'roughly two-thirds of a group of neurotic patients will recover or improve to a marked extent within about two years of the onset of their illness, whether they are treated by means of psychotherapy or not'. In a more extensive study, he concluded that psychotherapy was unessential to recovery: 'We have found that neurotic disorders tend to be self-limiting, that psychoanalysis is no more successful than any other method, and that in fact all methods of psychotherapy fail to improve on the recovery rate obtained through ordinary life-experiences and non-specific treatment.'[25] Some have challenged these findings, claiming that they were not sufficiently controlled to be considered scientific. Whether or not these criticisms have weight, Eysenck's studies served as a gauntlet challenging others to closely examine the claims of psychotherapy.

Suffice it to say that the invitation to validate the effectiveness of psychotherapy has not been met warmly by psychologists. Some would argue that 'there are studies available to substantiate or refute almost any claim one would like to make'.[26] Others would assert that 'because the research results indicate a great deal of uncertainty about what to do, psychologists' expert judgement can do better in prescribing treatment than these results'.[27]

Whatever the arguments, their primary intention is defensive, to protect the Psychology Industry from the increasing number of studies which draw the value of psychotherapy into question. For instance, in a review of therapy factors that account for significant client progress, Lambert found, as illustrated in Figure 2, that 'spontaneous remission' (improvement without treatment) accounted for 40 per cent, 15 per cent of the change resulted from placebo effects (the patients' expectation to get better no matter what was done), while a further 30 per cent improved as the result of common factors in the relationship such as trust, empathy, insight and warmth. Only 15 per cent of the overall improvement could be attributed to any specific psychological intervention or technique.[28] Based on this, one could conclude that 85 per cent of clients would improve with the help of a good friend and 40 per cent without even that. Many similar studies have supported the overall conclusion that most of the improvement attributed to psychotherapy is due to the general effects of talking to a warm, kind person and the effect of just naturally eventually feeling better anyway. White found that 55 per cent of therapeutic effects can be attributable to 'therapeutic rituals' which maximize positive expectations in all therapies.[29]

FIGURE 2

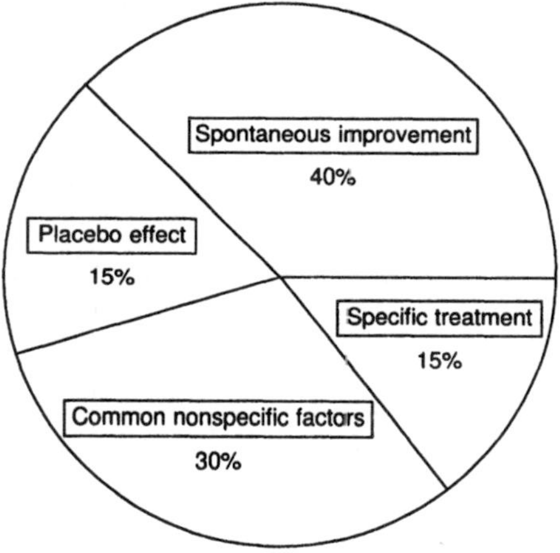

Many others have questioned the process of investigating the benefits of psychotherapy when the term merely serves as a rubric for a disparate group of treatments. Eysenck spoke of this when he described psychotherapy as 'a mishmash of theories, a huggermugger of procedures, a gallimaufry of therapies, and a charivari of activities having no proper rationale, and incapable of being tested or evaluated'.[30]

Such a concern has led some to suggest that the 15 per cent or so of change attributed to psychotherapy might be higher with some specific forms of treatment. However, Orlinsky and Howard concluded that there is no consistent evidence that any specific form of therapy produces better results than any other, whether it be individual or group therapy or family counselling, or short- compared to long-term treatment.[31] Similarly, studies have shown that the length or intensity of treatment has no appreciable effect on the improvement of clients[32] and that, despite loud arguments for long-term therapy, most change occurs in the first ten sessions.

Despite Orlinsky and Howard's conclusion, APA's Clinical Division Task Force[33] constructed a list of 'empirically validated treatments', including such approaches as:

- Behaviour therapy for headache, irritable bowel syndrome, female orgasmic dysfunction, male erectile dysfunction, enuresis and encopresis.
- Cognitive behaviour therapy for chronic pain, panic disorders, depression and generalized anxiety.
- Exposure treatment for post-traumatic stress disorder and phobias.
- Family education programmes for schizophrenia.
- Systematic desensitization for simple phobia.

The criteria for inclusion is at least two good studies showing the therapy to be better than a 'pill or psychological placebo or another treatment',[34] or equivalent to an already established treatment. In endorsing these approaches, the Task Force admits that they 'do not control for so-called non-specific factors like expectancy of change and contact with a supportive professional'.[35] While acknowledging this serious weakness, it identifies its current goal to 'move forward on a broader EVT list' rather than address the accuracy.

Almost immediately, this list has generated a new business enterprise: books, manuals, and training programmes are appearing with claims of being 'proven effective for improving clinical outcomes'.[36]

TherapyWorks® from The Psychological Corporation is a sophisticated example which claims that its 'programs have proven effective for improving clinical outcomes of specific disorders'.

Whether one agrees with their criteria or not, one thing that is noticeable is the absence of the 'talking cures' that focus on emotions and memories, which are used with the majority of Psychology Industry clients.

If the type, length and intensity of therapy generally have no significant effect on clients' improvement, one would hope that at least the therapist's training does. To examine this, Strupp and Hadley randomly assigned thirty clients with neurotic depression or anxiety reactions to either university professors who had no background in psychology or psychotherapy, or to professionally trained and accredited psychologists.[37] They found that the professionals were no more effective than the untrained professors, as assessed on a number of measures of clients' functioning. The only difference was that those treated by the professional therapists showed a bit more optimism; nevertheless, it failed to show any effect on their symptoms or functioning.

Other studies of therapist experience and psychotherapy outcome have similarly concluded that the level of experience of professional therapists is unrelated to their efficacy,[38] that accuracy in professional judgement does not improve with experience, and that paraprofessionals can be just as effective as well-trained professionals.[39]

These results fly in the face of the Psychology Industry's insistence that specialized training justifies higher fees. To counteract these findings, the APA has stated that it is 'important, perhaps imperative, that psychology begin *to assemble a body of persuasive evidence* bearing on the value of specific educational and training experience'.[40] In other words: we believe it works, we need it to look as if it works, so let's get numbers to make it look as if it works.

To provide support, an early 'meta-analysis' by Smith and Glass is often cited.[41] Instead of looking at the effect of therapy on individuals, meta-analysis looks at its summary effect in independent studies. In this case, the results of 375 outcome studies were considered with the conclusion that an individual who undergoes psychotherapy has a 2 to 1 chance of getting 'better' as compared to a person in the control group. However, the research has several flaws. 'Better' was not consistently defined; individual researchers determined their own meaning of 'better', often relying on clinicians' subjective ratings of improvement. While reporting this 66 per cent chance of being better off after therapy, the analysis fails to address the remaining 33 per cent, leaving it unclear whether they remain the same or get worse.

Since the intention of treatment is improvement, most studies have evaluated the positive effects, assuming that, at worst, psychotherapy is benign. However, some have considered negative change. A study compared students in encounter groups (with competent therapists) to students not in groups. After treatment, 57 per cent showed positive change and 29 per cent were neutral, but 14 per cent showed negative change. Six months after therapy, 46 per cent were still showing positive gains, 32 per cent were neutral, 21 per cent showed negative change. At first glance, this might suggest that the therapy was harmful. But a comparison to the all-important control group reveals that the change was similar in both groups, with 'negative change' occurring for some members of both groups. Therapy had not protected clients from getting worse but it could not, in this case, be held responsible for it.[42]

However, the results of the Cambridge-Somerville Youth Study, particularly relevant in this victim-oriented era, do indicate that therapy can be held responsible. In evaluating the effectiveness of a project designed to prevent delinquency in underprivileged children, 650 boys of six to ten years old were randomly divided into two groups with equal chances of delinquency. One group received individual therapy, tutoring and social services; the other received no services. The treated boys rated the project as 'helpful' and the counsellors rated two-thirds of the group as having benefited. However, the researcher, Joan McCord, followed the boys over time looking at effects on criminal behaviour.[43] The results showed little difference in terms of the number of crimes, but the counselled group committed significantly *more* serious crimes. A thirty-year follow-up showed the same pattern and revealed that, in terms of alcoholism, mental illness, job satisfaction and stress-related diseases, *the treatment group was worse.* McCord summarizes the results as ''More' was 'worse': the objective evidence presents a disturbing picture. The program seems not only to have failed to prevent its clients from committing crimes . . . but also to have produced negative side effects . . .'

McCord identifies three factors which may contribute to the harmful effects: *encouraged dependency, false optimism* and *externalized responsibility*; all of which are likely effects of many services promoted now by the Psychology Industry. She suggests that: 1) through therapy, the psychologists might have fostered a dependency among the boys, rendering them less able or inclined to cope with life's problems on their own; 2) 'the supportive attitudes of the counsellors may have filtered reality for the boys, leading them to expect more from life than they could receive'; and 3) counselling may have taught the boys that they were not responsible for their behaviour because it was a consequence of their underprivileged childhood experiences – an external cause to blame.

As one might expect, these conclusions evoked a response from psychologists: 'McCord's view is literal and simplistic. It lacks an appreciation of the intrapsychic processes that are effected by treatment . . . the consistently positive subjective reports of the treatment groups about their experiences must have some pervading impact on their lives today.'[44] In other words, if the boys say it is so, then it must be so, and you can't question it; a response now echoed by the Psychology Industry about its 'victims'.

McCord's study is not alone in its conclusions of harm. Ditman studied three groups of alcoholics who had been arrested and charged with alcohol-related offences. These individuals had been assigned by the court to either AA, an alcoholism clinic, or a nontreatment control group. A follow-up found that 44 per cent of the control group were *not* re-arrested, compared to 31 per cent of the AA group and 32 per cent of those treated in a clinic;[45] those that received treatment did worse than the untreated. 'Not one study,' Peele asserts, 'has ever found AA or its derivatives to be superior to any other approach, or even to be better than not receiving any help at all . . . every comparative study of standard treatment programs versus legal proceedings for drunk drivers finds that those who received ordinary judicial sanctions had fewer subsequent accidents and were arrested less.'[46]

Such findings are not rare. Robert Spitzer, of the New York Psychiatric Institute, comments that 'negative effects in long-term outpatient treatment are extremely common',[47] and the researchers Truax and Carkhuff state that 'the evidence now available suggests that, on the average, psychotherapy may be harmful as often as helpful, with an average effect comparable to receiving no help'.[48]

These studies serve as examples of the *psychiatrogenic* (therapist-caused) or *psychonoxious* (harmful to mind) damages that may result from therapy. For instance, psychologists often assume that the expression of emotion, 'getting it all out', is therapeutic and consequently they encourage 'ventilation' as an integral aspect of therapy. However, in a study of seven-year-old boys, those who were rewarded by approval for punching a doll were far more aggressive when they competed against other children later. Letting, or getting, it out actually increased the level of hostility, showing that 'rewards in therapy (approval) heighten the likelihood of subsequent violence'.[49]

Bergin acknowledges this risk when he writes:

> it now seems apparent that psychotherapy, as practised over the last fifty years, has had an average effect that is modestly positive. It is clear, however, that the average group data on which this conclusion is based obscured the existence of a multiplicity of processes occurring in therapy, some of which are known to be either unproductive or harmful.[50]

Hans Strupp estimates that one in ten patients is a psychonoxious victim of psychotherapy.[51]

Adding dramatic weight to this concern. Loftus and her colleagues reported the results of a preliminary study investigating a number of 'outcome effects' of therapy focused on repressed memories, and the costs involved:

> In 1990, Washington State permitted individuals to seek treatment under the Crime Victim Act if they claimed previously repressed memory for childhood sexual abuse. From 1991–1995, 670 repressed memory claims were filed. Of these, 325 (49%) were allowed.
>
> In the study, a nurse consultant (LP) reviewed 183 of these claims. Of these, 30 were 'randomly selected for a preliminary profile.' Some of the findings of this analysis are reported here. The sample was almost exclusively female (29/30 = 97%) and Caucasian (29/30 = 97%), with ages ranging from 15 to 67 yrs with a mean of 43 yrs.
>
> The women (and one man) saw primarily Masters level therapists (26/30 = 87%), although 2 saw a Ph.D., 2 saw an MD, and 6 saw a Master's level therapist in conjunction with an MD. The first memory surfaced during therapy in 26 cases (26/30 = 87%).
>
> All 30 were still in therapy three years after their first memory surfaced. Over half were still in therapy five years after the first memory surfaced (18/30 = 60%).
>
> Prior to memories, only 3 (10%) exhibited suicidal ideation or attempts; after memories, 20 (67%) exhibited suicidal ideation or attempts. Prior to memories, only 2 (7%) had been hospitalized; after memories, 11 (37%) had been hospitalized. Prior to memories, only 1 (3%) had engaged in self-mutilation; after memories 8 (27%) had engaged in self-mutilation.
>
> Virtually all the patients (29/30 = 97%) contended they had been abused in satanic rituals. They claimed their abuse began when they were, on average, 7 months old. Parents and other family members were allegedly involved in the ritual abuse in all cases (29/29); Most remembered birth and infant cannibalism (22/29 = 76%) and consuming body parts (22/29 = 76%); The majority remembered being tortured with spiders (20/29 = 69%). All

remembered torture or mutilation (29/29). There were no medical exams corroborating the torture or mutilation.

The sample of (mostly) women was fairly well educated, and most had been employed before entering therapy (25/30 = 83%), many of them in the health-care industry (15/30). Three years into therapy, only 3 of 30 (10%) were still employed. Of the 30, 23 (77%) were married before they entered therapy and got their first memory; within three years of this time, 11/23 (48%) were separated or divorced. Seven (23%) lost custody of minor children; all (30/30) were estranged from their extended families.

Whereas the average cost of a mental health claim in the Crime Victim Compensation Program that did not involve repressed memory was $2,672, the average cost for the 183 repressed memory claims was dramatically higher, $12,296.[52]

Although Loftus states that this does not 'prove' that therapy made these individuals worse, in a subsequent article she states that the results are alarming and the implications sufficiently serious to warrant further investigation into the harmful effects of repressed memory therapy.[53] She is not alone in this concern. Lief and Fetkewicz, after studying retractors of abuse accusations, write:

> As we collect more and more data on the types of therapies involved in recovered-memory therapy, we cannot avoid the conclusion that this is bad therapy . . . Patients get sicker instead of better, and huge sums of money are spent for years of therapy based on the erroneous assumption that the recovery of memories of sexual abuse in childhood is 'a healing process.'[54]

Subsequently, Washington State became the first to require corroboration of recovered memories in order to provide compensation in cases based upon them – an effort tantamount to defunding it, since documentation of corroboration is lacking for memories 'recovered' in therapy.[55]

If psychotherapy can be dangerous, then why do people still believe that therapy is safe and effective and seek it out in large numbers? The answer appears to be found in several interacting factors:

1) psychologists have a view of what constitutes a good patient and selectively choose these people, thus hedging their results;
2) 'good therapists' are judged by their personal characteristics rather than by their professional abilities; and
3) years of experience and opinion are wrongly equated with expertise and knowledge.

A 'good patient' has come to be known in the industry as a YAVIS, a person who is Young, Attractive, Verbal, Intelligent and Successful; in contrast to the HOUND, who is Homely, Old, Unsuccessful, Non-verbal and Dumb. Others have described the ideal patient as psychologically minded, reasonably intelligent, anxious, verbal and *not very sick.*[56] Kottler puts it this way: 'those who are trusting and disclosing, who have acute problems, no severe personality disturbances, and who are willing to accept responsibility for their growth, are going to do well in practically any form of therapy with almost any practitioner.'[57] In examining over 100 evaluation studies, Luborsky could find no special benefit of any treatment method but what he did note was that 'successful' treatment was tied to the patient's mental health at time of treatment: the studies 'indicate that the healthier a patient is to begin with, the better the outcome'. Thus, in this respect, the good patient is one who doesn't need to be a patient at all and for whom any problem or anxiety is likely to dissipate on its own anyway.

The other important patient characteristic repeatedly identified is *suggestibility* (or *gullibility*).[58] Hans Strupp identified that the best outcomes of treatment are found in those who are open to the suggestions of the therapist as to how to think, what to feel, how to act and what to believe.[59] By conforming to the psychologist's theories and belief system, experiencing emotions and memories as suggested by the therapist, the patient is seen to be improving. The selection of good patients is similar to the selection of subjects by a

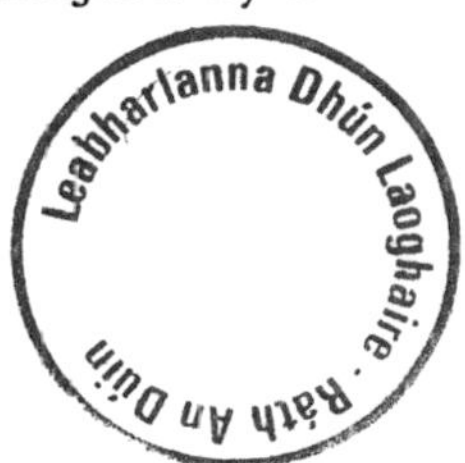

stage hypnotist: get interesting, attractive people who are suggestible, able to follow direction, want to comply and like attention.

For the 'good therapist' designation, it would seem that two characteristics are important. The first is that the psychologist must exude an aura of warmth, attentiveness, kindness, caring and trust; be 'a genuinely nice person'.[60] The other quality of this goodness is 'power'. Kottler, in describing what he called *The Compleat Therapist*, writes: 'it hardly matters which theory is applied or which techniques are selected in making a therapy hour helpful . . . What does matter is who the therapist is as a human being – for what every successful healer has had since the beginning of time is charisma and power.' He continues:

> Perhaps more than any other single ingredient, it is power that gives force to the therapist's personality and gives weight to the words and gestures that emanate from it. It was the incredible power that radiated from the luminaries in our field that permitted them all to have such an impact on their clients . . . nobody would have listened to them if not for their energy, excitement and interesting characteristics that gave life to their ideas.[61]

A similar expression of therapist worship is expressed by Guy in *The Personal Life of the Psychotherapist* when he writes that, with an outstanding therapist,

> there is a resultant transcendence which enables these special individuals to accomplish the 'impossible thing' . . . whether in session or on vacation, the fully integrated therapist constantly shares his or her senses of perspective and world view. A personal passion for psychic wholeness is incorporated into nearly every encounter, not because of an uncontrolled drive, but due to a genuine sense of mutuality and caring.[62]

If these self-perceptions of therapists are indicative of the common image of the 'good therapist', then it can be seen how they presume to act as experts in the absence of demonstrable expertise and to pronounce their effectiveness in the absence of evidence. They don't even attempt a systematic application of scientific principles. Instead, they base their practice on 'trained intuition' and 'clinical judgement' which allow them to transcend scientific principles and ignore the research findings.[63] In many ways, it becomes an enthralling dance of the patient and therapist, each responding to the moves and sways of the other and each believing that they are getting somewhere together. But when the music stops, the dance is over and therapy is finished, the most likely conclusion is that they aren't much further ahead, aside from one being a little (or a lot) poorer while the other is a little (or a lot) richer.

Playing the Numbers Racket

In the world of evaluation, it is exciting to discover a study that 'proves' that an approach of the Psychology Industry is effective. Such was the response to a study reporting the usefulness of psychotherapy in reducing medical utilization.[64] VandenBos summarized the results thus:

> [The researchers] found that persons with identifiable emotional distress, . . . made significantly higher than average use of both in-patient and out-patient medical facilities. When these emotionally distressed individuals received psychotherapy, their medical utilization declined significantly compared to that of a control group of matched emotionally distressed health plan members who did not receive psychotherapy. Significant declines in medical utilization were seen in the period following the completion of the psychological intervention and these remained constant. No additional psychotherapy was required to maintain the lowered level of utilization. It would, thus, appear that the costs of providing psychotherapy may be 'offset,' in part or whole, by cost savings resulting from lowered medical utilization.[65]

This was exciting because it demonstrated the effectiveness of psychotherapy in a study balanced by a control group and it provided strength to the economic and business approaches of the Psychology Industry. However, when playing the numbers racket, some numbers are better than others, and some data is sometimes better than all the data. A number of similar studies claim similar significant decreases in medical services following psychotherapy (as suggested by the right side of Figure 3).[66] But, as Schlesinger, Mumford and Glass point out, 'we can not take this conclusion at face value' for several reasons.

> Most of these studies present the psychotherapy group on what might be called 'relative time,' that is, the time series is constructed with the zero point at the time when each person in the psychotherapy group entered psychotherapy. But the control group is presented on 'absolute time.' The distinction is this: 'One month pre-therapy for the psychotherapy group might be January 1, 1975, for one person and August 15th, 1957, for another. In the control group all the people are on the same calendar time. Concern with what might, at first, seem a minor methodological problem derives from the likelihood that a person who seeks psychotherapy voluntarily does so in response to some felt need.[67]

Given that the emotional distress which creates this need might be accompanied by medical symptoms, it is reasonable to suspect that the time of beginning psychotherapy might also be a 'peak time of medical utilization', well above the individual's usual level (as indicated on the left side of Figure 3). Thus, the medical utilization would naturally decrease from the more severe level to one closer to the mean. This tendency is a statistical way of stating the common expression that when things are bad, things have got to get better; that is, move towards the average. Figure 3, a compilation of data from eleven studies, shows just this effect: the medical utilization for the psychotherapy group was far above their average as indicated by the level in years prior to therapy, and well above that of the control

FIGURE 3

EFFECTS OF PSYCHOTHERAPY ON MEDICAL ULTILIZATION

SYNTHESIZED AVERAGE OF ELEVEN ARCHIVAL TIME-SERIES EXPERIMENTS

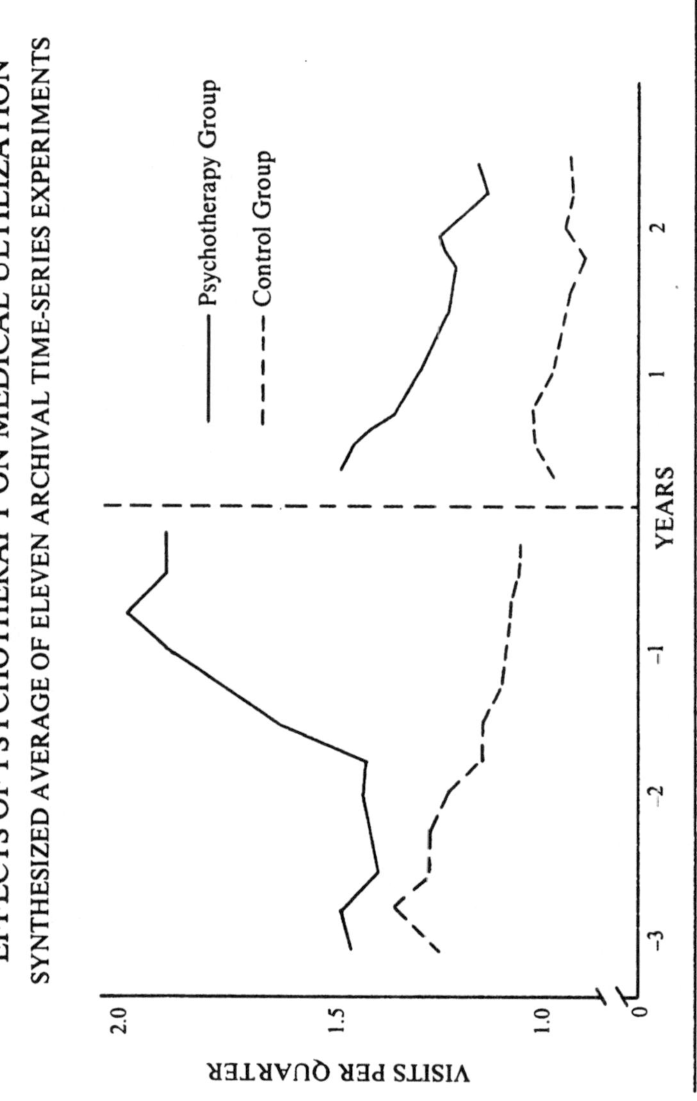

Synthesized findings of archival time-series experiments aggregated across 11 studies

group (left half of Fig. 3). Thus, it could have been predicted that the levels would drop to a level closer to the average. And it could also be assumed that this lower level, which is more typical of the person's usual utilization, would last with or without psychotherapy. If, at the same time, the person enters psychotherapy, it would be natural, although completely erroneous, to assume that the change is due to psychotherapy. Even the control (non-psychotherapy) group shows some regression towards the mean, with a smaller reduction. Schlesinger and his colleagues offer the following comment:

> Since the tendency of these methodological flaws is to inflate the apparent effect of psychotherapy on medical utilization, it is risky to take the integrated findings of these 11 studies at face value . . . a conservative conclusion would be that the likely influence of psychotherapy on reduction of medical utilization lies somewhere between 0% and 14%,[68]

far below that implied by VandenBos's earlier statement which claims dramatic effectiveness and cost savings. Another study of this 'offset effect' even found that psychological treatment 'boosted the overall care utilization and charges . . . above those of patients treated solely by their physicians . . .'[69] And Fraser, in cautioning that 'all that glitters may not be gold', points out that this medical offset effect may 'give deceptively positive results which may eventually undermine psychology's credibility with health providers'; a consequence that he attributes to the 'increased pressure for all psychologists to "sell" their services to an increasingly cost-conscious market'.[70]

It would appear that, in the case of health-related services, the involvement of psychologists increases the overall cost, while it provides them with additional income.

Science Fiction

. . . a great deal of what passes as attested theory is little more than speculation, varying widely in plausibility.[71]

In reflecting on his professional life, a former APA president, Paul Meehl, writes: 'Some things have happened in the world of clinical practice that worry me in this respect. That scepsis, that passion not to be fooled and not to fool anybody else, does not seem to be as fundamental a part of all psychologists' mental equipment as it was a half a century ago.'[72]

Some psychologists and users alike fool themselves into believing that they have great understanding of the causes of emotional problems, while others believe they have discovered a new and revolutionary cure. Others grasp hold of the pseudoscience because it seems to explain the unknown and calm the mind. As one psychologist put it: 'Science is a way to make people feel more comfortable by allowing them to explain things that they don't understand. In this way it compares to Greek mythology and modern religion.'[73]

But a number of these acclaimed therapies have turned out to be useless or worse. Biofeedback, popular in the 1970s, for instance, advocated that by gaining control over the autonomic nervous system, one could master one's state of being, both physically and mentally. It assumed that learning to 'produce' alpha waves, a type of brain wave which appears when people are relaxed, would cause people to be relaxed and gain control. Lacking supportive evidence, this presumption was then stretched so that claims were made that biofeedback could cure sexual disorders and deviance, muscle paralysis, migraine headaches, back pain, phobias, and even serve as a means of male contraception.[74]

Wrapped in the aura of science, biofeedback sessions took place in laboratories with white-coated professionals, physiological monitoring and printouts of brain, heart, muscle and skin functioning. Experts claimed that they could cure problems in a shorter period of time, persisting with these assertions despite research that showed unambiguously that these techniques did not work. This science was fiction, its explanations highly imaginary and its results fantasy.

Science fiction, whatever its focus, evokes intrigue by blending the known, the believable and the fantastic. From its starting point of 'what is', it travels into the realm of the 'what if'. Whether it begins with the submersible and goes 20,000 leagues under the sea, or with a space mission and becomes Star Trek, it merges science with fantasy, fact with fiction.

As a means of manufacturing victims, the Psychology Industry frequently delves into the world of 'what if', creating its own science fiction. Take for example the work of John Mack, a professor of psychiatry at Harvard University, who writes about his diagnosis and treatment of victims of 'alien abductions' in UFOs.[75] In his own version of the slippery slope, Mack begins with the regrettable fact that non-alien abductions occur and can have psychological consequences. Acknowledging that he is exploring at 'the margins of accepted reality', he then introduces the possibility that aliens and UFOs exist. Then, like a sleight-of-hand magician, he draws attention away from the 'what is' to the 'what if', wondering what might happen to victims while they are 'away' and what the later consequences, the 'universal properties of the abduction experience', might be. He states:

> abductees everywhere are compellingly drawn toward a powerful light, often while they are driving or asleep in their beds. Invariably, they are later unable to account for 'lost' periods of time, and they frequently bear physical and psychological scars of their experience. These range from nightmares and anxiety to chronic nervous agitation, depression, and even psychosis, to actual physical scars – punctures and incision marks, scrapes, burns and sores.[76]

With this theory and 'quite strict criteria of an abduction case', he proceeds not only to diagnose and treat abductees but also to assess the likelihood of an epidemic of UFO abductions: '2% of adults in the American population have had a constellation of experiences consistent with an abduction history . . . we believe that one out of every 50 Americans may have had UFO abduction experiences.'[77]

Acknowledging that indicators may not mean that an abduction has occurred, Mack says: 'a more serious difficulty in estimating the prevalence of abductions lies in the fact that we do not know what an abduction really is – the extent, for example, to which it represents an event in the physical world or to which it is an unusual subjective experience with physical manifestations.' And calling on recovered memory notions of repression, he continues:

> A still greater problem resides in the fact that memory in relation to abduction experiences behaves rather strangely . . . the memory of an abduction may be outside of consciousness until triggered many years later by another experience or situation that becomes associated with the original event. The experiences in a situation such as this could be counted on the negative side of the ledger before the triggering experience and on the positive side after it.[78]

By combining issues of abduction with pop beliefs in UFOs, then applying criteria unsupported by any independent research, constructing a diagnosis with psychological and physical consequences, Mack creates a problem which necessitates specialized psychological treatment. To support this, he weaves in the popularized concepts of sexual abuse and the controversial idea that memories reported in therapy or under hypnosis are true. With regard to memories he states that 'thinking of memory too literally as "true" or "false" may restrict what we can learn about human consciousness from the abduction experience'.[79] In other words, the experience is true beyond any question of whether the reported memories are true. Nowhere does he, nor could he, provide any independent scientific evidence for his science fiction.

For many, the whole notion can be dismissed as science fiction or nonsense. But Mack's reasoning is not unlike that applied to ritual abuse and day-care child abuse. In each instance, the psychologist claims to have special abilities to identify people who have been abused. 'It's so common that I'll tell you within 10 minutes, I can spot it as a person walks in the door, often before they even realize it,' said the on-air psychologist of the programme 'Good Morning America', maintaining that 'probably one in four women and one in eight men, have been incested'.[80] Based on clinical case examples rather than empirical studies, it is argued that these memories have been hidden from consciousness and retained somewhere in the unconscious where they continue to create psychic disturbances resulting in addictions, relationship difficulties, aggression and violence, passivity and dependence, and physical illness. The only help is psychological treatment to recover memories of the past; to acknowledge, accept and nurture the injured 'child within'; and to confront (and avenge) the wrongs and the wrongdoers.

Those supporting this approach believe that memory is historically accurate. The forensic hypnotist and psychologist Martin Reiser writes: 'the mind is like a video tape machine in that everything is recorded, perhaps at a sub-conscious level, and stored in the brain but available for recall under hypnosis.'[81] In the 1950s a neurosurgeon, Wilder Penfield, demonstrated that if a particular area of the cortex is electrically stimulated, patients could experience spontaneous flashbacks of old, apparently (though never proven) forgotten memories. It is now argued that Penfield's work proves that all memories are stored in the brain and can be retrieved and that psychological techniques can have the same power as Penfield's electrical probe, to discover memories. It is also presumed that the memory system functions from birth in the same way that it does throughout adult life. For example, a respected clinical hypnotherapist claimed to be demonstrating 'hypnotic regression' when he suggested to a woman that she go back to the time of her birth and describe her experience. She described the delivery room, the bright lights, the attending staff (identifying some by name), the cold air and the welcoming response of her mother. The hypnotist proceeded to affirm her recollections ('That's right! That's good!'), persuading her to accept the event and to see herself as wanted and loved. At no time during or after the session did he caution her that she might be imagining and that it might not be a true record of the events.

What scientific research does show is that memory is basically a reconstructive process; that remembrances are put together from partial memory traces and are remembered in such a way as to meet the needs or demands of the moment. Moreover, memory is dependent on what is first perceived. If something is not seen then, it can't be remembered later. The woman describing her birth experience didn't know that newborns have a fixed visual focal length and can't see more than 18 inches. She didn't know that she would not have seen, let alone known by name, who was in the delivery room. Without this knowledge, she responded to the psychologist's leading questions by constructing artificial memories based on information available to her as an adult. As the ability for visual perception changes after birth, so too does the child's ability to think, resulting in further changes in the style and content of memories. 'The fact is that no matter how the process of memorizing during infancy is measured, there is clear proof that it is far below the efficiency of that of the older child or adult,' stated the Social Science Research Council.[82] 'Tests of recognition, memory pictures, rote memory regularly show that human memory has proved to be poor at the earliest level and to increase by a fairly constant rate to a later period.' Memories of the past, particularly of childhood, are quite unreliable, since they mix and become confused with fantasies, information gained from other sources and at other times of life, and the suggestions or influences in one's immediate life. As Peter Wolfe writes in challenging the validity of reconstructed memories: 'The clinical reconstruction of early childhood experiences deals with the subject's present view about his past, and not with the discovery of archeological artifacts that have been buried.'[83]

If adult recollections of childhood are unreliable, perhaps at least children's reports of recent events are more dependable. Again the True Believer phenomenon becomes evident as child therapists and abuse experts make simplistic statements such as 'Children don't lie about sexual abuse!' and 'How would they know about such things [i.e. sexual acts] if it had not been done to them?' An interesting study involving anatomically detailed dolls sheds some scientific light on these claims. Forty three-year-olds were questioned in their paediatrician's office after receiving an annual medical examination. Half the children received a genital examination involving gentle touching of the buttocks and genitals, while the other group did not. Immediately after each individual check-up, a researcher, using an anatomically detailed doll, asked the children to show, using the doll, how the doctor had touched their buttocks and genitals (either a leading or misleading question). Results showed that the children were very inaccurate: for those who had a genital examination, 45 per cent denied touching when asked directly, and the error level increased to 57 per cent 'when these children manipulated the dolls to demonstrate the genital exam', because some children falsely showed that the doctor had inserted a finger into the anal or genital cavity. Accuracy was also low for children who had not received a genital examination: 42 per cent of their responses included false claims that they had been touched when asked 'Did he touch you?' and 38 per cent of their responses on the dolls showed that the doctor had touched their genitals or anal region. The children also demonstrated a number of other sexualized behaviours during the interview, some using other props in a sexual manner on their own bodies or on the dolls.[84] This illustrates that not only are children very inaccurate in reporting sexual touching but also that the rate of false positives (reports of touching in the absence of any) is comparable to the level of false negatives (failure to report what did happen).

Some psychologist claim that the memory is impaired because some events of childhood are so traumatic that the mind represses them from consciousness, but retains them unconsciously, where they continue to affect adult life. However, repression, a Freudian concept, has no scientific support and much of what is purported to be examples of repression can more easily be understood through normal forgetting, remembering what one wants to remember, or 'infantile amnesia' which, Sears writes, 'is apparently a biological trick of an undeveloped memory system, not a Freudian twist of unconscious repression'.[85] Despite this lack of supporting evidence, many psychologists interpret the failure to remember events of childhood as indicative of repressed memories of child abuse. To wonder about possible abuse is considered to be indicative of such memories 'slipping through' to consciousness. Bass and Davis write: 'If you think that you were abused and your life shows the symptoms, then you probably were.' And they continue: 'so far no one we've talked to thought she might have been abused and then later discovered she hadn't been.'[86] Such circular arguments are among the catch-22s of the Psychology Industry's reasoning. Defying objective validation, they argue that if one represses, then one doesn't remember, so that if one doesn't remember, then one must be repressing memories; and if you think or wonder about abuse, then you are a victim, and if you don't, then you are denying the fact. A speech to new AA members demonstrates this: 'If you think you have a problem, or if you think that you are an alcoholic, I assure you that you are. You wouldn't be thinking about it and you wouldn't be here if you weren't an alcoholic.'[87]

Having achieved this level of absurd thinking, psychologists can lead their patients into the belief of abuse, the pursuit of memories and the creation of their own science fiction.

Caveat Emptor: Buyer Beware

The aim of science is not to open the door to everlasting wisdom, but to set a limit on everlasting error.

Bertolt Brecht

In many ways, fact has been replaced with fiction, and knowledge with beliefs. The 'science of psychology' has become the 'business of psychology', persuading the public that psychotherapy offers the solution to their problems. But does it?

Two recent independent studies evaluated this claim with very different results. The first, the *CR* Study, concluded that:

1) Psychotherapy works: 'our groundbreaking survey shows that psychotherapy usually works.'
2) Long-term therapy makes a difference: 'Longer psychotherapy was associated with better outcomes.'

The second, the FB Study, concluded that:

1) Psychological services may not work: 'Clinical services . . . very effectively delivered . . . in a higher quality system of care that were nonetheless ineffective. A very impressive structure was built on a very weak foundation.'
2) Long-term treatment isn't better: 'More is not always better.'

One can imagine which results the Psychology Industry chose to publicize and promote. Obviously, psychologists want to tell everyone about the first and hide the second. A critical look reveals what information is being selectively concealed.

The CR Study

CR stands for *Consumer Reports*, an American magazine that talks about how satisfied consumers are with their vacuum cleaners and toasters. In November 1994 it reported on a 'candid, in-depth survey' of its readers regarding their satisfaction with psychotherapy in an article entitled: 'Mental health: Does therapy help?'[88] Martin Seligman, the 1998 president of the APA and the consultant to the project, described the results in a companion article in the flagship journal of the APA as sending 'a *message of hope* for other people dealing with emotional problems' and as establishing a '*new gold standard*' for the evaluation of psychotherapy effectiveness.[89]

Before accepting this endorsement, attention must be given to how the survey was done and how the results were interpreted.

The *CR* report and Seligman's article were based on the results of a supplement to the 1994 annual automobile survey sent to 180,000 subscribers. Readers were asked to respond 'if at any time over the past three years [they had] experienced stress or other emotional problems for which [they] sought help from any of the following: friends, relatives, or a member of the clergy; a mental-health professional like a psychologist, counsellor, or psychiatrist; your family doctor; or a support group.' In the usual style of *CR*, it was a consumer-satisfaction survey. It did not ask respondents objective, factual questions such as how much alcohol they drank, how often they fought with their spouse or considered suicide before going for help as compared to after. Nor did it seek independent verification of the self-reports. Instead it asked readers how much better they felt and how much they thought therapy had helped them. From these responses came the 'convincing evidence that therapy can make an important difference'.

Seligman admits that the response rate was 'rather low absolutely'; and *CR* describes it as 'very low' when compared to its other surveys. (A similar article on physicians received 70,000 responses, over 24 times larger than in this survey.[90]) Despite the broad invitation to readers, only 7,000 (3.9 per cent) responded to the mental-health survey; of these, 4,000 (2.2 per cent) reported seeing a mental-health professional, family doctor or attending a support group; the remaining 3,000 (1.6 per cent) had talked to a friend, relative or cleric. *CR* chose to ignore the experience of this latter comparison group of 3,000, and attended to only the 4,000, with particular emphasis on the 2,900 (1.6 per cent) who saw mental-health professionals.

This small sample, consisting mostly of middle-class, well-educated and predominantly female individuals, with a median age of forty-six, was not at all representative of the general population. Seligman dismisses this problem by 'guessing' that it is representative of those 'who make up the bulk of psychotherapy patients', never giving further thought as to what this may mean both for the data and about the upper-middle-class nature of psychotherapy.

In most other cases, such a low return rate and skewed population sample would have rendered a study invalid, not acceptable for publication and therefore not warranting any further analysis or comment. But these inherent problems did not stop *CR*, Seligman or the

Psychology Industry from proceeding to draw sweeping conclusions about the worth of psychotherapy. In reference to their two claims, this is how they 'analysed' their meagre data.

DOES THERAPY WORK?

Seligman's authoritative answer is that 'the overall improvement rates were strikingly high across the entire spectrum of treatments and disorders in the *CR* study'.

Both the *CR* article and the subsequent marketing material from APA claim that nine out of ten people were helped by psychotherapy. But for psychotherapy to work, one needs people with problems. Such is not the case here. Over half of the respondents (58.2 per cent) said that they felt 'so-so', 'quite good' or even 'very good' before treatment. Seligman apparently doesn't scratch his head at this point and wonder whether these people are 'therapy junkies'. Rather he assesses them as 'being sick' and not knowing it, referring to them as '"sub-clinical" in their problems' and falling 'one symptom short of a full-blown "disorder"'. However, from a common-sense, non-psychologized perspective, these people might be considered normal, okay or even in great shape. Perhaps, for them, psychotherapy was more recreational than therapeutic. And, if so, how does one really know whether treatment is even appropriate, let alone whether it works?

To add further to the confusion over effectiveness, Seligman states that 64 per cent of those receiving six months or less of therapy reported that their problems were resolved. However, his own chart indicates that, when averaged across disciplines, only 30 per cent of the people reported that treatment 'made things a lot better' with respect to their specific problems. One is left wondering how is it possible that 64 per cent reported that their problems were resolved when only 30 per cent said that their problems were improved? Both numbers are far below those claimed by APA and *CR* when they say that psychotherapy helps nine out of ten people, leaving one wondering about the extent of inaccuracies and misinformation.

Whatever the percentage is, *CR* and Seligman assume that the reported improvement in people's feelings while they were seeing a mental-health professional is attributable to the psychotherapy. But can this assumption be accepted? Think about this. If people are given an antibiotic and their colds go away in a few weeks, can it be concluded that the antibiotic cured the cold? It can't, because most people naturally get over a cold in a week or two. So too do the stresses and emotional upsets in life usually abate over time. As Eysenck demonstrated, over time, people show comparable improvement with or without treatment. Moreover, as Dawes points out, if

> people enter therapy when they are extremely unhappy, they are less likely to be as unhappy later, independent of the effects of therapy itself. Hence, the illusion that the therapy has helped to alleviate their unhappiness, whether it has or not. In fact, even if the therapy has been downright harmful, people are less likely to be as unhappy later as when they entered therapy.[91]

To determine whether therapy was really effective for those in the *CR* survey, a comparison group is needed of people with similar problems who did not receive treatment. While a formal control group is not available, a comparison group does exist composed of those who spoke to friends, relatives and the clergy. Both groups described their emotional state at the time they filled out the survey, which would have given some indication of the effect of time. However, *CR* was unwilling, when repeatedly asked, to provide any further information or clarification or even to reveal whether these groups were similar. They claimed that these data were proprietary and would not be analysed or released. While Seligman said that he, too, would like to see the data, on another occasion he expressed assurance that 'there was nothing of substance to be found there'.

We are left wondering about these concealed data. If, in fact, professional treatment was superior to lay help, would not *CR* and Seligman want the public to know this? And if it was not more effective, would not the *CR*, and the APA, have the responsibility to inform 'consumers' that people are no more satisfied by paid services than by ones that are free?

IS LONG-TERM PSYCHOTHERAPY BETTER?

The handling of the data with regard to this question can best be addressed by comparing two graphs. The first one, from Seligman's article, visually suggests that the answer is obvious; that the longer the therapy, the better the outcome. Seligman, in fact, stated: 'long-term therapy produced more improvement than short-term therapy. This result was very robust . . .'

However, a closer look reveals that the vertical axis that measures 'improvement' is truncated, beginning at 190, not 0, where one would expect it to start. The visual effect leads one to presume that the change is small at the beginning and significantly greater over time.

FIGURE 4

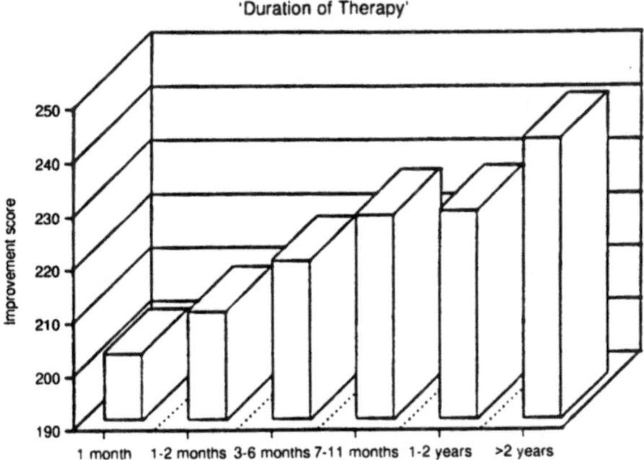

However, if this chart is accurately redrawn, this dramatic effect disappears, showing that most of the 'improvement' (83.4 per cent) actually takes place in the first month; and further treatment of up to two years and more contributes less than 17 per cent. Seligman

FIGURE 5

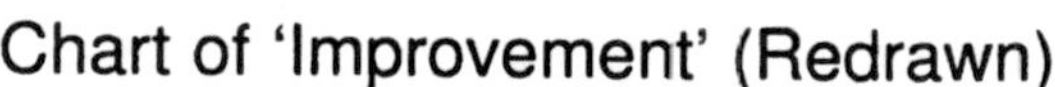

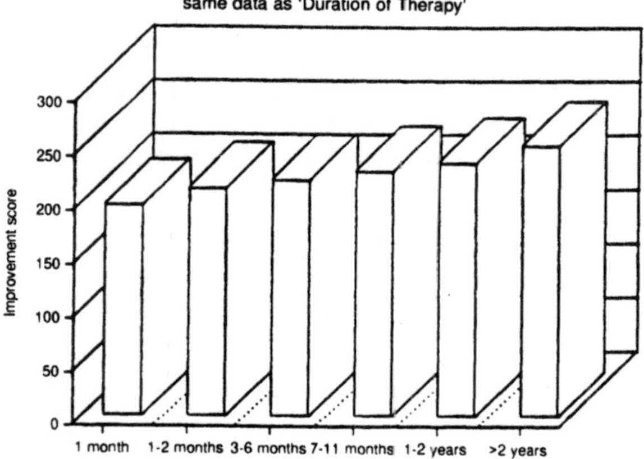

himself states that the left bar 'approximates no treatment'. Hence it would seem that most problems improved with little, if any, treatment.

The FB Study

FB stands for the Fort Bragg Demonstration Project, funded at a cost of $80 million of public funds.[92] Cast in such glowing terms as 'a national showcase' and 'state of the art', this study was intended to show that 'a continuum of mental health and substance abuse services is more *cost-effective* than services delivered in the more typical fragmented system'.[93] While the *CR* survey suffered from serious methodological problems and continues to be criticized for its numerous flaws, the only criticism lodged against the FB Study was that it had not been replicated, a weakness which was overcome by the results of a similar study in Stark County, Ohio, with similar findings at the six-month and two-year follow-ups.[94]

The FB Project offered inpatient and outpatient services to more than 42,000 child and adolescent dependents in the Fort Bragg catchment area for more than five years. This group from middle- and lower-middle-class families was representative of the majority of the children who are covered by private health insurance. And most importantly, unlike the *CR* survey, the FB Study evaluated treatment effectiveness and outcome, not relying merely on reports of consumer satisfaction. Instead of questionable retrospective self-reports, it relied on independent psychometric measures systematically taken both during and after treatment.

As such, the project provided what Leonard Bickman, its senior researcher, describes as 'a rare opportunity to examine both costs and clinical outcomes in a careful and comprehensive evaluation of the implementation of an innovative system of care' which psychologists predicted would increase accessibility to treatment, improve results through individualized case management, and reduce overall costs.

However, what it found was that, despite better access, greater continuity of care, fewer restrictions on treatment and more client satisfaction, the cost was higher and the clinical results no better than those at the comparison site: not at all what the Psychology Industry had either expected or wanted! Even though users expressed satisfaction about their treatment, there was no evidence of effectiveness, supporting the opinion that 'satisfaction' is not a measure of effectiveness.

In summarizing the significance of these results, Bickman and others drew the main following conclusions.

One: the assumption that clinical services are in any way effective might very well be erroneous.

Citing the lack of clinical outcomes as 'the most unanticipated finding', Bickman states that 'these results should raise serious doubts about some current clinical beliefs' about the effectiveness of psychological services. He continues: 'although substantial evidence for the efficacy of psychotherapy under laboratory-like conditions exists, there is scant evidence of its effectiveness in real-life community settings (i.e. outside of the research setting).'[95]

While some have asserted that therapy works because '50% of

the children improved the year after intake, as defined by losing a diagnosis',[96] there is no evidence that these children would not have improved over this time period without the expense of psychological services. Moreover, in the Stark County replication study, it was found that a group of children whose parents reported that their children received no mental-health services improved at the same rate as the children who received many services.[97] This discouraging conclusion is supported by another major study by Bickman's colleague Bhar Weiss, who carefully examined the effect of two years of traditional child psychotherapy as it is typically delivered in outpatient settings. What he found was not the expected benefits but rather no effect at all.[98]

Two: longer treatment results in higher costs without corresponding significant results – more is not better.

The Psychology Industry argues strenuously that involved clinicians are the best judges of what treatment should be provided and for how long. Yet, the Fort Bragg data shows that what psychologists call their 'experienced clinical judgement' is not cost-effective and leads to a higher proportion of children being in treatment longer. 'Six months after starting treatment, 41% at the Demonstration site were still receiving services compared to 13% at the Comparison site,' even though most of the limited change that did occur was evidenced in the first six months with greatly diminishing returns after that time.

Stating that 'more is not always better', Bickman reports taking a much closer look at the data to determine whether there was a dose-response relationship between number of outpatient visits and outcomes. He could not find any such relationship. 'One visit or 50, the children improved at about the same rate.'[99] He attributes the excessive use of long-term therapy to the unlimited access of psychologists to funds. 'The Demonstration costs were much higher ($7,777 treated child) than the Comparison ($4,904/treated child) . . . The costs of treating the average child were higher because of longer time spent in treatment, greater volume of traditional services, heavy use of intermediate services, and higher per-unit costs.' Feldman agrees, stating that 'the study demonstrates that in an unmanaged system of care when services and benefits become rich so do providers'.[100]

The Seligman and *CR* stance that 'longer is better' and that the public is suffering when limits are imposed on the length of therapy falters in the face of the data from the Fort Bragg Study. As Hoagwood, from the National Institute of Mental Health, states, referring to this project, 'the belief that simply providing more services will lead to improved outcomes has been shown to be delusional,'[101] reminding us of A. E. Housman's comment of a hundred years ago: 'the pursuit of truth in some directions is even injurious to happiness, because it compels us to take leave of delusions which were pleasant while they lasted.'

The ominous cautions about the effectiveness of psychotherapy have been echoing throughout the halls of the Psychology Industry for decades. In 1961, Hobart Mowrer succinctly wrote: 'There is no shred of evidence that psychoanalyzed individuals benefit from the experience.'[102] A similar message was voiced by Morris Parloff, of the National Institute of Mental Health (NIMH), in 1979. After reviewing a large number of studies of psychotherapy, he paraphrased the proverbial farmer and said: 'The best I can say after years of sniffing about in the morass of outcome research literature is that in my optimistic moods I am confident that there's a pony in there somewhere.'[103] Not so optimistically, Robyn Dawes summarized his findings in this area of psychotherapy research in 1994, writing 'that there is no *positive* evidence supporting the efficacy of professional psychology. There are anecdotes, there is plausibility, there are common beliefs, yes – but there is no good evidence.'[104]

What is the reaction of the Psychology Industry? These studies and conclusions are not touted, as the *Consumer Reports* one is, in the APA public education campaign. It is unlikely that they will affect the practices or change the beliefs of those within the industry for, although they are well designed, well implemented, well analysed, and produce results that are about as clear-cut as can be imagined, they don't support the current claims of the Psychology Industry. 'In the end,' as Sechrest and Walsh put it, 'what it comes down to is whether professional psychology is going to be guided by its dogma or its data'[105] or, put somewhat differently, whether it will use science to guide its action or misuse science to sell its products.

Seligman's own warning to consumers, though he may now choose to ignore it, seems worthy of repeating:

> Making up your mind about self-improvement courses, psychotherapy, and medication . . . is difficult because the industries that champion them are enormous and profitable and try to sell themselves with highly persuasive means: testimonials, case histories, word of mouth, endorsements . . . all slick forms of advertising.[106]

In the world of the Psychology Industry, the concept of 'caveat emptor' bears special importance because 'science' is a particularly powerful sales pitch. As Frank Farley, a past president of APA, says, 'the science side of psychology is in selling ourselves in [the] market.'[107]

4

The Business of Psychology

The demand for psychotherapy keeps pace with the supply, and at times one has the uneasy feeling that the supply may be creating the demand . . .

Jerome Frank

'Don't confuse me with the facts' might very well be the slogan of an industry that is not deterred by research that questions the usefulness of its services. When Neil Jacobson wrote: 'It is not uncommon for therapists to keep clients in therapy long after it is obvious that little or no progress is being made,'[1] the APA president, Robert Resnick, responded: 'Such opinions are, of course, just that. Our rebuttal should be outcomes research and practice patterns. As psychologists like to say, the data will speak for itself.'[2]

The data indeed speak; they confirm that psychology's claims are exaggerated, its benefits dubious. But the Psychology Industry proceeds undaunted, measuring its success not by research findings but by satisfied customers. Science is merely an aspect of its marketing. Resnick says: 'The lack of plentiful research on the effectiveness of psychotherapeutic interventions has hampered *our ability to thrive* . . .' Nowhere does he acknowledge the already plentiful research that fails to support psychotherapy effectiveness.

It is difficult for the public, conditioned to trust and respect professionals, to consider that the Psychology Industry may have a bottom line based on profit rather than on clients' welfare. It is troublesome to think that a business that offers understanding and hope to others can have its attention focused on its own interests. And it is hard to imagine that its success rests on insinuating itself into everyone's personal life.

While some might consider this growth of the Psychology Industry to be evidence of a profound national need of epidemic proportions, it can equally, and more accurately, be seen as an indication of the highly effective marketing techniques used to generate the demand required to meet the ever-increasing supply of psychologists. As Jerome Frank observed:

> Ironically, mental health education, which aims to teach people how to cope more effectively with life, *has instead increased the demand for psychotherapeutic help.* By calling attention to symptoms they might otherwise ignore and by labelling those symptoms as signs of neurosis, mental health education can create unwarranted anxieties, leading those to seek psychotherapy who do not need it. The demand for psychotherapy keeps pace with the supply, and *at times one has the uneasy feeling that the supply may be creating the demand.*[3]

While it is difficult to get an accurate reading of the total number of practising psychologists, estimates are that the number in the United States has risen twenty-fold since 1970. The picture of saturation[4] becomes more dramatic when one considers that licensed psychologists constitute only one quarter of those who refer to themselves as psychologists and less than 5 per cent of the estimated total number of psychologists as defined in this book. Using this broader definition, there is one psychologist for every 250 people in the United States.

Not only has supply kept up with demand, it has far exceeded it, creating the need for new 'products' and new markets for psychological services. This is occurring at a time when there are dramatic changes in the marketplace; old markets are drying up and new ones have to be established. Zilbergeld's 1983 claim that 'virtually everyone can get counselling at a price he can afford to pay' no longer holds. Today, psychologists of different persuasions vie for the limited health dollars and openly compete for clients.

And as attention has shifted from 'health and welfare' to 'law and order', so too has that of the Psychology Industry. Whereas the secret of success for a psychologist once was to develop a professional association with a physician or psychiatrist, it now is to develop a working relationship with law enforcement or the legal profession.

In light of the economic and social changes in society, the Psychology Industry has to create a new marketing plan and business approach along with an ever-expanding array of new products and services.

Selling the Psychology Industry

. . . actually, no less than the entire world is a proper catchment for present day psychiatry (and psychology), and psychiatry need not be appalled by the magnitude of the task . . .
Our professional borders are virtually unlimited.

Howard Rome, past president,
American Psychiatric Association[5]

Essential to the success of most industries is their ability to market themselves. Although some naive members of the Psychology Industry would like to believe that psychological problems exist in and of themselves, creating their own demand for services, such is not the case. Some may criticize those who openly promote their services. However, few acknowledge that giving free public lectures or interviews to the media on psychological topics can serve the same promotional function.

This marketing takes the three-pronged approach of psychologizing, pathologizing and generalizing. Variations on this approach can be seen whenever psychologists talk to clients or to each other; when they lecture, give interviews, testify in court or appear in the media; in the books and articles they write; and in the representations and petitions that they make to government and funding agencies.

Psychologizing

In 1914, *Good Housekeeping* magazine published an article proclaiming that 'the amateur mother of yesterday' would be replaced by 'the professional mother of tomorrow'. No longer were women to rely on their maternal instincts, the wisdom passed down through generations, or the advice and support of family, friends, and other members. American mothers were being persuaded to turn for advice to professionals, who at that time were heavily influenced by Freud's theories.[6] Child-rearing began to be considered a psychological task that required expert guidance if it was to be done properly. Not long after the article, the behaviourist John Watson applied behavioural theories to child-rearing, giving further strength to the psychologized notion that professionally directed parenting could create successful children while avoiding the pitfalls leading to problem children.

From then, psychologists of all persuasions began to lay claim to child-rearing as one of their areas of expertise as they psychologized life, from 'the birth experience' to 'the death experience', into a complex array of psychological theories and processes. Taking the words of David Smail seriously when he writes regarding psychology that 'anything people can do for themselves is the waste of an opportunity to make money',[7] the Psychology Industry has undertaken to psychologize all of life. Psychologists 'really do intend that all of life should be included in their sphere of influence'[8] and, to ensure that no one escapes, they have dissected life into a variety of phases and events, attributing to each some specific psychological importance. Events once handled by common experience or passed-down wisdom, and greeted with joy and happiness or sadness and regret, are now put under sterile psychological management. Millions of intelligent, educated people have been persuaded to rely on paid professional advice.

Whether it is an aspect of superiority or arrogance, professionalism or paternalism, psychologists consider themselves to be the experts. 'Our social problems are all human problems,' as George Albee puts it; 'and we [psychologists] are the experts on this.'[9] Resonating this view and embellishing it, Frank Farley, the 1994 APA president, writes that psychology 'may be in the process of re-inventing itself as the primary discipline in the solution of humanity's major problems . . .'[10]

Although this attitude now pervades society, it is by no means new as evidenced in the activities of the Freudian and behavioural child-rearing experts at the beginning of the twentieth century. Parenthood is replete with examples of psychologizing and its effects, ranging from how to interpret children's nightmares to quelling their fears or administering discipline. In 1994 a father was charged with assault after spanking his five-year-old daughter in public after a talk and a warning failed to stop her misbehaviour. Psychologists spoke up against the father, saying that 'spanking does not make sense because it fails to address the underlying reason for a child's behaviour. At the same time it spawns a host of adverse reactions, anything from aggression and violence to fear of speaking and acting later in life.'[11]

Curiously, at the same time, legislation was being proposed to hold parents legally as well as financially responsible for the misbehaviour of their children, again based on the psychologized assumption that the illegal activities of children were due to incompetent parenting and inadequate discipline. Sometime earlier, Tom Hansen of Boulder, Colorado, had used this idea to sue his parents for $350,000, charging that his mental health had been impaired by 'inadequate parenting'. The claim was based on allegations that his father made him dig weeds in the yard when he had caught his son smoking marijuana.[12]

In the psychologized world of child-rearing, the amateur parent is clearly at risk not only of *feeling* guilty but also of being *found* guilty. The only thing that parents can feel confident in is that the standard of today will change tomorrow, the psychological truth of today will soon be called nonsense. As Gross writes:

> The creation and dissemination of knowledge on how to raise children now appears to be one of the greatest academic hoaxes of our times. Judging from the accumulated evidence, it appears probable that the intelligent, intuitive parent knows as much, or more, about child care as the child educator, the parent–child expert, the psychologist, the social worker or the psychiatrist.[13]

However, the psychiatrist Jack Westman does not agree. He proposes an accreditation process in which parenting would be restricted to individuals who are at least eighteen, have completed a certified course in parenting and have signed a pledge not to neglect or abuse their children. Westman would treat unlicensed parents like unlicensed drivers, taking their newborns from them until they have met the necessary requirements.[14]

Childhood has always been a popular target for psychologizing since it is so amenable to being abstracted into systems of stages and phases, each with its own school of experts. There are experts in infant bonding and infant stimulation, in moral, religious, social, psychological and intellectual development, in early childhood education, for underachievers and overachievers, in conduct disorders and shyness, in learning disabilities and cooperative play.

But psychologizing has taken over virtually every aspect of human existence. There are psychological experts in death and dying, obesity and eating disorders, being married and being single, sexual pleasure and dysfunction, being fired and being successful, midlife crisis and growing old, child care and elder care, and so on.

Nowhere, however, is the entrepreneurial psychologist more evident today than in the courtroom. As early as the 1970s, the APA expressed the 'expectation that in the future forensic psychologists *will roam confidently and competently* far beyond the traditional roles of psychologists'.[15] This prediction is being realized. A 1995 article by APA states that 'diversification is a viable form of self-preservation . . . Psychologists may still get a steady stream of clients paying out-of-pocket, but not enough to replace third-party payments . . .' And it continues: '*Forensics offers broad opportunities for psychologists* with the appropriate training. Their expertise can be used for custody evaluations, divorce mediation or expert trial testimony.'[16]

Health care used to be the lucrative arena of choice for psychologists; now it has clearly been replaced by the legal system. This was made explicit at a 'psychology and the law' conference at Villanova Law School where participants agreed that psychology 'is poised to grab a more prominent role in law after years on the sidelines'.[17]

In 1884, the New York Court of Appeals stated that 'twelve jurors of common sense and common experience' would do better on their own than with the help of hired experts, 'whose opinions cannot fail to be warped by a desire to promote the cause in which they are enlisted'.[18] Despite this, it wasn't long before psychological experts began to appear in courtrooms. In the famous trial of Leopold (aged nineteen) and Loeb (aged eighteen), who were accused of killing a thirteen-year-old boy, psychological evidence formed the major defence. Clarence Darrow, the defence lawyer, noted: 'For the first time in a court of justice, an opportunity was presented to determine the mental condition of persons accused of crime, according to the dictates of science and modern psychiatry, without arbitrary and unscientific limitations imposed by archaic rules of law.'

Thus began the long and well-established tradition of psychologists consorting with lawyers to the point where 'the pursuit of truth, the whole truth and nothing but the truth has given way to reams of meaningless data, fearful speculation, and fantastic conjecture. Courts resound with elaborate, systematized, jargon-filled, serious-sounding deceptions that fully deserve the contemptuous label used by trial lawyers themselves: junk science.'[19]

Huber notes that 'junk science is matched by what might be called liability science, a speculative theory that expects lawyers, judges, and juries to search for causes at the far fringes of science and beyond'. He continues: 'Sometimes . . . the cheapest point of control will be at quite some distance from the scene of the accident. The search for the cheapest possible control must inevitably lead out to the edges of scientific knowledge.'[20] And psychologists have responded in sympathy, tracking back and back, searching the fringes of human experience and identifying causes which can serve either to relieve responsibility or to place the blame.

The psychologist Margaret Hagen, in *Whores of the Court*, writes:

> When the law welcomes the astrologer into the courtroom as possessing the same status as the astronomer; when the court listens to the priest with the same critical judgement it applies to the testimony of the physicist, then and only then will the testimony of clinical psychologists about the formation and functioning of the human mind in general or in particular individuals make sense as expert testimony. When the concept of expertise is itself debased to nothing more than personal opinion, then the clinicians should take the stand along with the rest of the opinionated. Why not? Until then, throw them out of the courts.[21]

An amusing variation on this suggestion was proposed recently by a New Mexico state senator (*opposite*)

VALIDATORS – THE TWENTIETH-CENTURY WITCH-PRICKERS

Just as the witch-hunts of centuries ago were controlled by the inquisitors who had the power to declare people as heretics, so now do psychologists control the uncovering of abuse and trauma and have the power to identify perpetrators.

In discussing the witch-hunts of England, Christina Hole writes: 'One of the most terrifying features of the general witchcraft belief was the fact that no one knew for certain who was, or was not, a witch.' And she continues: 'The most deplorable by-product of the general fear of witches was the professional witch-finder',[22] whose pay depended on the number of witches discovered. The witch frenzy spawned a new profession of 'witch-prickers', some of whom were physicians and some of whom were 'common prickers'. Their practice was to stick a pin into the skin of anyone suspected of being a witch and, based on the degree of pain or bleeding, they either confirmed those as witches or recommended further 'examination' by an ordeal of immersion in water – never acquitting

WIZARDS OF ID

'When a psychologist or psychiatrist testifies during a defendant's competency hearing, the psychologist or psychiatrist shall wear a cone-shaped hat that is not less than two feet tall. The surface of the hat shall be imprinted with stars and lightning bolts.

Additionally, the psychologist or psychiatrist shall be required to don a white beard that is not less than eighteen inches in length and shall punctuate crucial elements of his testimony by stabbing the air with a wand.

Whenever a psychologist or psychiatrist provides expert testimony regarding the defendant's competency, the bailiff shall dim the courtroom lights and administer two strikes to a Chinese gong.'

From an amendment proposed in March 1995 by Duncan Scott, a New Mexico state senator, to a bill addressing the state's licensing guidelines for psychologists and psychiatrists. According to Scott, the proposal was intended to draw attention to the rise of 'insanity pleas in criminal trials.' The amendment was approved by the state senate but was rejected by the New Mexico House of Representatives.

(Harper's Magazine, July, 1995, p. 16)

them. After the publication of the *Malleus Maleficarum* (*The Hammer of Witches*), the manual for witch-hunters, 'a class of men sprang up in Europe who made it the sole business of their lives to discover and burn the witches,'[23] and these lay-prickers along with physicians became the first recognized legal experts. 'The parliaments had encouraged the delusions [in witchcraft] both in England and Scotland, and by arming these fellow [prickers] with a sort of authority, had in a manner forced the magistrates and ministers to receive their evidence.'

Just as the power and prestige of these prickers rose with the increasing identification of witchcraft, so too has the influence and income of psychologists risen with the increasing reports of abuse. Like their predecessors, these twentieth-century prickers have gained status and built businesses on identifying invisible signs. While it is questionable whether witches ever existed, it is not disputable that child and adult abuse does occur. And it is upon this basis that the industry of 'assessing' and 'examining' has been built; some practitioners even referring to themselves as 'validators'.

In validating the reports of children, play-therapy techniques involving anatomically accurate dolls, interviews and physical examinations are often relied on. With adult accusers, clinical interviews, hypnosis, and behavioural lists are generally the basis for determinations and expert testimony. Despite the prominence these validating psychologists have achieved, their techniques remain highly questionable. Research has shown that children provide their adult interviewers with the type of information they think the adult wants, and that when this is coupled with leading and misleading questions, play therapy or the use of dolls, the effect is to tell the interviewer whatever he or she expects.[24] The reliance on physical examinations to provide evidence of sexual abuse, which has been used subsequently in the conviction of many people, has proven to be so unreliable that the American Medical Association has issued specific guidelines. The use of check lists and 'consistent with sexual abuse' reasoning has similarly come under criticism because of the vagueness of the behavioural items which would allow almost anyone to qualify as a victim. Hypnosis, often employed as a memory-enhancement procedure, is also questioned, and in some American states, the use of hypnosis bars individuals from testifying because of the significant effect of hypnotic suggestion and the unreliability of resulting memories.

Validators have also appeared in recent years among those who treat and assist people with severe developmental disabilities such as autism. Using a method known as 'facilitated communication', which involves providing physical support as the handicapped individual types out messages on a keyboard, at least five dozen allegations have been made leading to charges of abuse against parents, teachers and other care-givers.[25] This is occurring despite controlled research which shows not only that the people with these disabilities are unable to respond accurately, but also that the responses they appear to give are actually those of the assistants, the validators.[26]

Given this, one might assume that there would be limited reliance on validators and that they would have to be specially trained and highly qualified professionals. But such is not the case, for many

> are self-styled 'therapists' who have absolutely no training at all, even in related disciplines . . . Many of these ill-qualified and incompetent individuals take 'courses' in which they are trained by people of questionable qualifications . . . Some of these therapists have also crept into the sexual abuse field where they serve as not only evaluators but therapists as well. *Sex abuse is a 'growth industry'*.[27]

They have found a niche and are exploiting it to their own advantage.

Beginning in the early 1980s, a series of infamous large-scale or community-wide child-abuse cases have grown out of this industry. Among the best known is the McMartin case, one of the costliest trials in American history. Kee MacFarlane, the now discredited interviewer of the children in that case, testified emotionally before the US Congress in September 1984 about powerful conspiracies of sexual predators who appear to be running pre-schools across the country. She compared the sexual pillage at these facilities to nuclear warfare and called for community disaster planning to combat it. Two weeks after this testimony, Congress doubled its funding of child-protection programmes. MacFarlane's programme was itself the beneficiary of huge federal and state grants.[28]

While validators claim to identify victims, they are, in fact, manufacturing victims: both fabricated abuse victims and victims of false allegations. Like the ecclesiastic epidemiologists of witchcraft who benefited from a high rather than low incidence of this witchcraft, the psychologists who seek to identify victims and to persuade public opinion that a social problem is worse than previously thought, have a vested interest in inflating the numbers.

Pathologizing

In a world in which everything has two meanings, the common one understood by most and the psychologized one open only to the understanding of psychologists, it is not surprising that virtually every aspect of life can become pathology. At one time, treating serious mental illness was the major responsibility of psychologists, but now it is only a minor activity. The Psychology Industry prefers to 'abolish the hospital only to make the whole world a hospital'[29] and everyone a patient. In so doing, it actively sets about to convince people that even minor discomforts are symptomatic of deeper, more severe problems.

The formula for pathologizing, drawing its structure from traditional medical practice, is to define what is normal, make a diagnosis, recommend a psychological treatment, and state the expected outcome with and without treatment.

For instance, Zimbardo and Radl, promoting shyness therapy, state:

> our primary concern is to help you to minimize the effects *[the treatment]* of shyness *[diagnosis]* that may keep your children from reaching their full potential as human beings *[prognosis with treatment]*. Even when children are only moderately shy *[implication*

> *that shyness is abnormal]*, they still miss out on valuable social experiences. And, when shyness is really severe, living in that psychological prison can ruin a life *[prediction with no treatment]*.[30]

To assess pathology, a concept of normality must be established. But what is this psychological state called 'normal'? Ruesch and Bateson argue that normal is whatever doesn't appear in the lives of psychotherapy patients. They believe that 'since the [psychologist's] attention is focused on deviation, and since he has little or no training in normal psychology, he tends to construct a hypothetical norm by averaging the exact opposites of those features he sees in his patients.'[31] So, if patients are unhappy, happiness must be normal; if patients are insecure, then security is normal; if patients are anxious, then calmness is normal. Normality, as Freud said, becomes 'an ideal fiction'.

While this may explain the popular view of normality as bliss, the Psychology Industry has gone even further in creating this illusion. Consider Marone, who in her book on learned helplessness, states: 'it is fear that begets the most intense feeling of helplessness. Fear of being alone, fear of being attached; fear of failure, fear of success; fear of change, fear of monotony; fear of living, fear of dying; the list is as endless as there are individuals in the world.'[32] One concludes from this that if fear leads to helplessness and helplessness is a pathology, then fear is abnormal. But, according to her, fear is experienced by everyone, so everyone has fear: fear is therefore normal and 'normal' is therefore abnormal. Such is the Psychology Industry's paradoxical and convoluted logic as it sets an absurd standard. It is the marketing of this form of 'normality' that sustains the Psychology Industry and creates victims, as fear, unhappiness, insecurity, sadness, anxiety, failure and so on become synonymous with psychological illness.

In promoting this fantasy of normality, the Psychology Industry forces people to consider themselves psychologically disabled. When once people were ashamed of being diagnosed, many are now eager and willing, provided that the label (1) explains and justifies their problems and behaviours, leaving them with little or no sense of guilt or responsibility, and (2) is socially acceptable, making them feel special and understood without feeling stigmatized.

Unsupported epidemiological claims have been made for countless pseudo-diagnoses, making them seem both legitimate and sufficiently prevalent to be acceptable. American examples include:

- 25,000,000+ are alcoholics.
- 80,000,000 suffer from co-alcoholism.
- 20,000,000 are gambling addicts.
- 30,000,000+ women suffer from anorexia or bulimia.
- 80,000,000 have eating disorders.
- 75,000,000 (30 per cent of population) are cigarette addicts.
- 50,000,000 suffer from depression and anxiety.
- 43,000,000 (⅓ of all women) are victims of PMS (premenstrual syndrome) or PPD (post-partum depression).
- 25,000,000 are love or sex addicts.
- 5,600,000 have been abducted by UFOs.
- 22,000,000 suffer from debilitating shyness.
- 66,000,000 are incest survivors.
- 10,000,000 suffer from borderline personality disorder.
- 36–48,000,000 are diagnostically addicted to work.
- 12,000,000 (5 per cent of all Americans) suffer from 'generalized anxiety disorder'.
- 200,000,000 suffer from the impostor phenomenon, a psychological syndrome based on intense, secret feelings of fraudulence in the face of success and achievement.
- 1,350,000/yr have post-traumatic stress disorder after a car accident.
- 4,200,000 women have developed PTSD after being sexually assaulted.

This incomplete list of possible diagnostic labels accounts for over 800 million Americans, more than three times the US population, supporting the Psychology Industry axiom that it is normal to be abnormal.

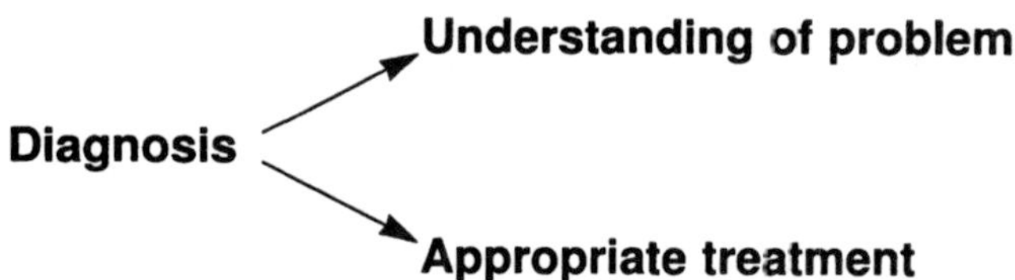

Traditionally in medicine, a diagnosis has served the dual purpose of determining the nature of the problem and indicating the appropriate treatment. However, in the Psychology Industry it is generally the case that the diagnosis is adjusted to fit the form of treatment offered by the assessing psychologist, and 'practice patterns indicate that psychologists most often use the treatments that they prefer, rather than the treatments that are tailored to patient needs'.[33]

Preferred Treatment ——► Preferred Diagnosis

Consider the following comment by Anne Wilson Schaef: 'I was toying with the idea that many of the categories found in the *DSM-III* fit much more readily under the rubric of addiction and co-dependence, and working with them with the tools of the Twelve-Step program and the deep process work not only was cheaper and easier, it was more effective.'[34] What she admits is that she takes the wide variety of psychological problems and redefines them as addictions, making her treatment, 'deep process work', the most suitable.

So often, in the Psychology Industry, the diagnosis is consistent with the treatment offered that one can only surmise that the psychologist's area of interest determines both the label and the treatment. This was intimated by Frank Pittman, who writes: 'psychotherapy involves applying the value system of the therapist to the dilemmas of the clients . . . his or her value system is more important to you than training, credentials, or even professional degrees.'[35] Sometimes, and probably not infrequently, the diagnosis simply becomes a catalogue number for insurance reimbursement, unrelated to assessment or treatment. As Pittman confesses: 'I sell them my time and whatever wisdom I have developed. If they expect their insurance to pay for it, I may apply a psychiatric diagnosis to them as well.'

Not only does the Psychology Industry use pseudo-diagnostic labels to create the market for treatment, it also uses 'fear appeal' to sell it. The *Dictionary of Marketing and Advertising* defines 'fear appeal' as 'advertising purporting to develop anxiety within the consumer based on fear that can be overcome by purchasing a particular item or service' as is done in 'selling fire insurance by depicting a burnt-out house'.[36] For the Psychology Industry, the burnt-out house is replaced by the psychological disaster that waits if one does not purchase help. Their attitude is evident in Zimbardo and Radi's earlier statement 'living in that psychological prison can ruin a life', or in that of Marcone: 'current research shows that this style of behaviour systematically sabotages the very core of an individual's ability to cope with the rigorous demands of living in the world today . . . The price of helplessness can range from producing minor inconveniences, to obscuring one's vision of major opportunities, to binding one to dangerous or abusive situations.'[37] These are the purported fearful risks of shyness and learned helplessness if left untreated.

Similar statements are made by the Psychology Industry with regard to most types of victim. Psychologists declare that psychological trauma 'is like being hit by a truck',[38] and that 'verbal abuse is *literally* dangerous to our health, in the same way that contaminated food and polluted water and toxic waste are dangerous'.[39]

But appeal to fear alone would not readily sell a product or service were it not for the complementary emotional image that is portrayed once one makes the purchase. For the home-owner, it is the peace of mind that comes from having purchased fire insurance. For the psychology consumer, the 'emotional appeal' is similar. Harris and Reynolds, trying to persuade parents to get therapy for their teenage children, write: 'When your teen comes home from a therapy session, you may notice attitudinal changes. Your youngster will be developing *greater self-esteem, improving confidence, and becoming more assertive and expressive.*'[40] And Marone, selling treatment for learned helplessness, describes the mastery-oriented individuals who 'create reality and alter the world to fit their conception of it'. She adds: 'For the benefit of us all, they demonstrate in living color that the world will yield to the creative and focused application of a committed psyche.'[41] For victims, the promise is not merely 'surviving' but 'thriving'; the goal is to achieve the 'optimal'. It's no longer all right to be just 'OK', one has to be 'perfect'; for 'no matter how free of disease or problems you are and no matter how well you are doing, it's not enough,' everyone could do better.[42]

When pathologizing is combined with the psychologized expert role, courtrooms become gold mines for the Psychology Industry. The following are examples of cases in which psychologists were paid to pathologize. (Numbers in parentheses indicate the *DSM-IV* classification code.)

- Battered-wife syndrome: In October 1998, a Canadian woman murdered her sleeping husband and escaped prison by offering uncorroborated claims that her actions were due to his abuse.
- Premenstrual syndrome: A jury in Liverpool, in December 1994, found a woman not guilty in the killing of her husband after she was diagnosed as suffering from PMS.
- Somatoform disorder (300.81): A Canadian university professor was ordered to pay his adult daughter £1,500 per month until he retires because she is unable to work due to a disorder that makes her focus on her physical disability.
- Clerambault–Kandinsky syndrome: A psychologist testified that Sol Wachtler, chief judge of New York State, charged with extortion and threatening to kidnap the teenage daughter of his ex-lover, 'was manifesting advanced symptoms of CKS', described as involving an irresistible lovesickness or 'erotomania'.
- Telephone scatologia (302.90): A psychiatrist argued that Richard Berendzen, forced to resign from the presidency of

American University after being arrested for making obscene phone calls, suffered from this paraphilia.

- Computer addiction: In Los Angeles, when a computer hacker pleaded guilty to theft after breaking into a corporate computer system and stealing software, the judge saw him as the victim of the insidious disorder of 'computer addiction', and sentenced him to treatment for this 'new and growing' impulse disorder.
- Attention deficit/hyperactivity disorder (314): Steve Howe, who received a lifetime suspension from baseball for an extensive series of cocaine violations, successfully fought the ban, arguing that he was a victim of ADHD, despite the fact that this diagnosis applies to children and Howe was thirty-four years old.
- Sleepwalking disorder (307.46): This diagnosis was used successfully in the 1980s defence of a Canadian man charged with the murder of his wife's parents, after he drove 15 miles across Toronto in the middle of the night to commit the act.
- Cultural psychosis: A defence lawyer in Milwaukee argued that a teenage girl charged with shooting and killing another girl during an argument over a leather coat suffered from 'cultural psychosis' which caused her to think that problems are resolved by gunfire.
- Reactive attachment disorder: A Denver woman, charged with beating her adopted two-year-old to death with a wooden spoon, defended herself by arguing that the child actually beat himself to death. The treating psychologist, Byron Norton, presented the theory that, owing to neglect and poor nurturing at infancy in a Russian orphanage, the child suffered from an 'attachment disorder' which caused difficulty in attaching to care-givers, resulting in a rage during which he inflicted the injuries on himself. The prosecutors called the definition 'pop psychology at best and voodoo at worst', but the judge ruled to allow the defence.
- A 'novel' disorder. The novelist Janet Dailey, whose romance books have sold over 200 million copies, acknowledged plagiarizing a rival's work, stating: 'I recently learned that my essentially

random and non-pervasive copying are attributable to a psychological problem that I never suspected I had. I have begun treatment for the disorder and have been assured that, with treatment, this behaviour can be prevented in the future.'

- Beanie Baby addiction. A woman who used stolen credit cards to 'feed her habit' for these stuffed toys received five years' probation on the condition that she doesn't touch her drug of choice: Beanie Babies.

Pathologizing, based on presenting an idealized and unachievable image of 'normal', and proceeding to label and treat people based on this abstraction, is a powerful factor in the marketing of the Psychology Industry.

Generalizing

In 1973, the Polsters wrote: 'Psychotherapists have recently glimpsed *the vast opportunities* and the great social need to extend to the community at large *those views* which have evolved from their work with troubled people.'[43] But what are 'those views'? In most cases, they involve two generalized concepts: *trauma* and *addiction*. If one person suffers from the effects of trauma after a vicious attack, or another develops a chemical dependency on alcohol, then maybe these terms can be indefinitely stretched to apply to many more people, even those who haven't even recognized that they are suffering and troubled. And what better way than to take a psychological term, popularize it through books, lectures, workshops and the media, and then apply it to a whole host of situations? Referring to this process as 'semantic inflation', Thomas Szasz noted that it 'has resulted in the transformation of the ordinary behaviours of ordinary persons into the extraordinary and awe-inspiring symptoms of mental diseases'.[44]

The situation in which the predicted trauma of hostages was generalized to compare to others' experience of divorce, a relative's death or a robbery, is but one example. Familiar concepts such as co-dependency, self-esteem and violence also illustrate this 'take-it-

and-run' strategy of the Psychology Industry which taps the 'vast opportunities' that the Polsters saw.

THE CO-DEPENDENCY EPIDEMIC

'Co-dependency' was coined to explain women whose lives were so intertwined with those of their alcoholic husbands that they were considered to be indirectly dependent on alcohol. Their lives were seen to derive meaning from their role of rescuer or nurse. But co-dependency is no longer restricted to alcoholism, it has been resculpted to apply to any problem associated with any addiction suffered by any family member or anyone close. This has served to expand the market to include families, friends, business associates and lovers; anyone who might seek help. And it has opened the floodgates to allow virtually every facet of life to become an addiction. Anne Schaef contends that 'an addiction is anything we are not willing to give up',[45] an interpretation that is supported by the following partial list of topics for invented addictions: sex, love, chocolate, shopping, religion, food, caffeine, gambling, computers, television, work, speed (i.e. moving fast), anger and fast food.

This generalizing of addiction spawned the recovery movement. It has given birth to a subsidiary industry that provides treatment for all those addicted to the addicts: those that are co-dependent. As Jeffers jubilantly proclaims: 'At last there is a Twelve Step program that benefits us all! You may never have had reason to attend any of the Twelve Step programs such as Alcoholics Anonymous (AA) . . . *But everyone in our society, including you and I, has reason to attend one of the newer Twelve-Step programs – Co-dependents Anonymous (CODA)!*'[46] Melody Beattie confirms this: 'Co-dependency involves our responses and reactions to people around us. It *involves our relationships with other people*, whether they are alcoholics, gamblers, sex addicts, over eaters, or *normal people*.'[47] Further redefined as 'a disease of loss of selfhood',[48] co-dependency can be applied to anyone who has ever felt that they have done something they didn't want to do because of someone else – a group that is estimated to consist of 96 per cent of the US population.

In creating this generalized concept of co-dependency, the Psychology Industry blends the original concept from the field of alcoholism with the passion and promise of religious revivalism, the medical concepts of disease and epidemic, and the victim-making process of externalizing cause and blame. According to co-dependency authors, it is a result of one or another form of child abuse, either physical, sexual, verbal or neglectful, which in turn has led to the self-neglect or self-abuse of co-dependency. Within this circle of logic, everyone becomes both a victim of his or her own dysfunctional family and of the 'universal problem of addiction'. Schaef asserts that 'when we talk about the addictive process, we are talking about civilization as we know it'.[49] Rome's prophetic words that 'no less than the entire world is a proper catchment' are coming true as millions of people search for psychological answers. One publisher of co-dependency books is reported to have said 'A lot of people are looking at why they're not happy'[50] and turning to co-dependency as a possible explanation.

Once co-dependency has been psychologized (equating external relationships and internal dependence) and then generalized ('millions are identifying themselves as co-dependents'),[51] it is a natural next step for psychologists to pathologize it, casting it in terms of disease. Consider Ricketson's negative prognosis: 'As you fall prey to addictions and continually living from a false self, *you will eventually break down under the strain.* Untreated co-dependency *invariably leads to stress-related complications, physical illness, depression, and death.*'[52] Such bizarre statements led Wendy Kaminer to note that the definition of co-dependency as 'bad and anyone can have it . . . makes this disease look more like a marketing device'.[53]

SELF-ESTEEM AS A PRODUCT

As diagnoses are being generalized, terms such as 'self-esteem' and 'violence' are being sponged into the overall fabric of society. Nathaniel Branden, author of *The Psychology of Self-Esteem*, wrote: 'I cannot think of a single psychological problem – from anxiety and depression, to fear of intimacy or of success, to spouse battery or child molestation – that is not traceable to the problem of poor self-esteem.'[54] It can be used both to explain problems and to describe the positive outcomes of psychological treatment. Remember Harris and Reynold's statement: 'When your teen comes home from a therapy session, you may notice attitudinal changes. Your youngster will be developing greater self-esteem, improving confidence, and becoming more assertive and expressive.'[55]

Self-esteem has become embellished to the point where lack of it is generally accepted as one of the major causes of personal and social problems, which must be directly addressed before people will change or social problems can be solved. As one psychologist wrote: 'every theory of mental health considers a positive self-concept to be the cornerstone of a healthy ego.'[56]

Such a belief led the California State Assembly to set up a task force charged with the mission of promoting self-esteem.[57] The legislature believed that raising self-esteem would reduce welfare dependency, drug abuse, teenage pregnancy and other social ills. The task force assumed that self-esteem was at the root of both good and bad behaviour and set about to 'determine that it [was] scientifically true'. In doing so, it generalized the view of self-esteem, attempting to show the causal connection to child maltreatment, academic achievement, sexual activity of teenagers, unwanted teenage pregnancy, crime and violence, welfare, alcoholism and drug use. The problem they encountered was that what they 'knew' to be true turned out not to be. The editor of the report admitted that 'one of the disappointing aspects of every chapter . . . is how low the association between self-esteem and its consequences are in research . . .'[58] But contradictory findings have never daunted the Psychology Industry. So, despite the admission that 'there is no basis on which to argue that increasing self-esteem is an effective or efficient means of decreasing child abuse', the report went on to recommend that 'policy interventions to reduce child abuse that involve increasing self-esteem should be encouraged and should include interventions at the individual, family, community and societal levels'.[59]

Janet Woititz, author of *Adult Children of Alcoholics*, showed a similar oblivious response when confronted about her research data which showed that children of alcoholics who attended Alateen had a lower self-esteem than those who did not attend. To deal with this, she explained:

> Thoughtful analysis of the data and an understanding of the alcoholic family pattern can help explain this result. Denial is a part of the disease both for the alcoholic and his family . . . This researcher suggests that the non-Alateen group scores significantly higher than the Alateen group scores because the non-Alateen children are still in the process of denial – they deny feeling badly about themselves.[60]

When an abstract psychological concept is generalized in such a way that it becomes a cultural mythology, it can be applied to all aspects of human life as either cause or consequence, whether it fits or not.

MARKETING THE THEME OF VIOLENCE

Violence would, at first glance, appear to be different from self-esteem; it seems real and brutal. Violence, however, actually serves as an excellent motif for Psychology Industry promotion. It plays to the current concern of society for law and order while serving to tap into public funds which, while being reduced in the health sector, are being increased for justice and policing. For instance, the APA Board of Professional Affairs identifies the 'application of psychological expertise to managing major social issues and changes such as violence' as a future role for psychological practice.[61]

Violence can refer to murder, assault, rape and physical abuse but, in this psychologized world, it can also mean 'any act that causes the victim to do something she does not want to do, prevents her from doing some things that she wants to do, or causes her to be afraid'.[62] Just as low self-esteem can be blamed for failure and disappointment, so too can violence, when broadly defined, be seen as the cause of problems for which an 'other' can be held responsible.

Despite statistics which show a dramatic decrease in violent crimes, violence, aggression and fear have become popular themes for psychologists to use in their marketing.[63] Ignoring the unfulfilled promises of the 1950s to eradicate crime, the Psychology Industry offers 'a message of hope' that, for instance, 'there is overwhelming evidence that [psychologists] can intervene effectively in the lives of young people to reduce or prevent their involvement in violence.'[64] This promise is made even though the same report acknowledges 'the lack of availability of outcome data on many existing youth violence prevention or treatment programmes'.

The psychologizing of violence leads people to believe that it is due to psychological causes, as demonstrated by the following statements made to the Canadian Senate in a debate on violence in society:

> I have never met a violent juvenile delinquent who was not abused as a child . . . Secondly, all of the criminals at San Quentin prison who have been studied had violent upbringings as children.
>
> All assassins, or individuals who have attempted assassinations in the United States during the past 20 years had been victims of child abuse: There is a 100 per cent correlation.
>
> If you look at the problem of sex murder . . . you find that they all come from broken families and suffered cruelty and brutality, usually at the hands of a woman . . . You see the pattern over and over again. There is cruelty to animals, cruelty to kids, and if a woman has beat up on you, then you are more likely to become a sex murderer.[65]

The implication is that violence is due to psychological factors and that psychologists are capable of understanding and doing something to eliminate it. Through fostering a culture of fear and contrasting it with the ideal of security, psychologists create for themselves a niche at the politico-cultural level by advising on issues of prevention and policy-making and proposing ways of identifying or treating perpetrators. For instance, one psychologist, using 'fear appeal', warns that 'only one to five per cent of sex offences are reported' and 'the next-door neighbour or community leader may well be an undiscovered paedophile'.[66]

Meanwhile, the APA task force on male violence against women, whose members were described as 'experts in different aspects of female-directed violence', declares that 'one in every three women will experience at least one physical assault by an intimate partner during adulthood' and '34 to 59 per cent of women are sexually assaulted by their husbands'.[67] Based on weak to nonexistent research, these claims exacerbate public fear.

Although this task-force report claims to have 'ways to curb violence', most of its recommendations were for further research. Specifically regarding intervention, it recommends 'encouraging treatment innovation' (presumably because current programmes are ineffective), 'enhancing practitioner knowledge of the history of traumatic victimization, routine screening for histories of victimization and validating women's experiences as part of clinical practice'; and it suggests that sensitivity training be provided to judges[68] and grants be established to create innovative techniques to increase arrests, prosecution and conviction rates in domestic violence cases. In other words, although psychologists want the public to view violence in psychological terms and psychologists as the experts, they possess no remedies.

While much of the Psychology Industry's attention is directed towards 'controlling violence' and identifying offenders, other psychologists, such as Judith Becker, president of the Association for the Treatment of Sexual Abusers, propose increased funding for the psychological treatment of offenders. As an example, Becker refers to the mass-murderer Jeffrey Dahlmer, whom she had evaluated for his 1992 trial, as 'a lonely soul who found sadistic control as his only escape from isolation', and whose 'cannibalistic compulsions may have been alleviated had he felt safe to seek help when his deviant fantasies began in his adolescence'.[69] Despite the view of many psychologists that such serious offenders are untreatable, and in spite of Dahlmer's own claim that none of her ideas made sense to him, Becker and her associates believe that funding should be provided to help 'offenders explore the origins of their sexual compulsions – which usually involves their own victimization – and explore more appropriate alternatives'.[70]

So, whether distorting statistics, making frightening statements or claiming unsupportable abilities to treat or prevent violence, the Psychology Industry persuades society of its powers. At the same time, it pathologizes those who have survived real violence. Psychologists' predictions that, although the incidents may have passed, the psychological effects are ongoing and may be long-term, have given rise to a plethora of government-funded victim-support services, staffed and directed by psychologists. The Psychology Industry has succeeded in creating the expectation of an 'emotional backlash'. However, one elderly woman, whose home was burgled in her absence, when offered professional help to deal with the trauma and fear she was presumed to be experiencing, said that the only help she needed was in cleaning up the mess.

While many might agree with her and concede that not all crimes cause psychopathology, most would probably assume that childhood sexual abuse inevitably requires psychological intervention. But such beliefs are not supported by research. No one doubts that serious abuse can have lasting effects; however, the assumption that it *always* leads to pathology seems inaccurate. For instance, Nelson found that, while 65 per cent of the female incest victims in her study did regard the experience as negative, 9 per cent were uncertain about their feelings and 26 per cent evaluated what had happened to them as positive.[71] Burgess and Hartman found, in a study of the consequences of sex-ring exploitation involving the abuse of children by one or more adults, that three quarters of those studied 'demonstrated patterns of negative psychological and social adjustment'[72] – the expected outcome. What is striking is the complementary finding that 25 per cent of these cruelly mistreated children appeared to be psychologically unharmed.[73] Levitt and Pinnell concluded, in their review of the research literature, that 'many victims – a sizable minority at least – do not suffer long-range harm. One possible cause of this finding is that father–daughter incest, the most virulent type, is far less common than sibling incest. Another inference is that children are more resilient emotionally than non-professionals like Bass and Davis believe.'[74] Whatever the reason and whatever the proportion, it is clear that not all are damaged victims.

If not all victims are psychologically harmed by violence, then what about those who only witness it? The Psychology Industry would have society believe that they too are victims. In 1995 Paul Bernardo was tried and convicted in Toronto, Canada, for the murder of two teenage girls, both of whom had been held captive, repeatedly raped, sodomized, beaten and eventually strangled. Videotapes, obtained by the police, were played to the jury showing the gruesome scenes. At the conclusion of the trial, jurors were asked to attend a two-day session to deal with their trauma, victims of having had to view the tapes. Interestingly, most refused.

Other psychologists have taken to altering the concept so that it includes insults and criticism. Suzette Elgin states that 'physical violence begins, 99 times out of 100, with verbal violence';[75] a claim which she later said was 'not intended as a "statistic"'. In the same generalizing vein, Catharine MacKinnon, a legal theorist, claims that she was raped by a book review. Carlin Romano, the book critic for the *Philadelphia Inquirer*, began his review of MacKinnon's book *Only Words* with a hypothetical proposition: 'Suppose I decide to rape Catharine MacKinnon before reviewing her book. Because I'm uncertain whether she understands the difference between being raped and being exposed to pornography, I consider it required research for my critique of her manifesto . . .' The effect according to MacKinnon was that of rape: 'He wanted me as a violated woman with her legs spread.'[76]

Another example of 'definitional ooze' can be found in the report of the US Secretary of Health and Human Services Donna Shalala that, according to a government-funded study, 'child abuse and neglect nearly doubled in the United States between 1986 and 1993'.

One odd thing about her claim is that no other sign points to such a dramatic increase in abuse or neglect. Fatalities arising from child abuse, for instance, held roughly steady.[77] Further examination reveals that 80 per cent of her 'increase' can be accounted for by the inclusion in the criteria of 'endangered children': those who were not actually harmed or neglected but 'in danger of being harmed according to the views of community professionals', those 'emotionally abused' by virtue of 'verbal abuse' or 'the refusal or delay of psychological care', or suffering 'educational neglect', involving the chronic failure to send a child to school. The apparent explosion of abuse can, more accurately, be attributed to the lavalike spread of redefinitions of abuse and neglect.

Thus, it would seem that, according to the Psychology Industry, one can be a psychological victim of violence whether the violence is experienced directly, witnessed, or watched on television or a movie, and regardless of whether it is physical, verbal or even imaginary. Like co-dependence and 'self-esteem', violence helps to increase the size of the pie for psychologists to slice up.

The Clothes Have No Emperor

In 1993, Jeff Blyskal wrote in a popular magazine:

> Last February, I decided to become a psychotherapist.
>
> I found a comfortable office in the East Fifties for a mere $875 a month. IS Furniture Rental was willing to outfit the place in traditional style, with plenty of rich burgundy tones – cherry desks, medical-file cabinets, couch, even oil paintings – for only $335 a month.
>
> The cost of business/appointment cards would come to $70; the phone, installed, would cost $621.81; a month long radio-ad campaign (60-second spots, four times a day) would reach a quarter-million listeners for only $2,000.
>
> So for just $4,000, I could have become a professional healer – with absolutely no training, credentials, or licence.[78]

Blyskal didn't hang up his shingle but he could have because, contrary to public belief, in most North American jurisdictions there is nothing to stop such a scam.

Since the option is open to anyone, the first step in becoming successful is to imply competence. Many rely on their academic qualifications and, if possible, use them to achieve licensing or gain restrictive certification. For most, a doctorate provides the licence to 'roam freely', declaring expertise as they go.

Lacking doctorates and licences, a common way for some to obtain credentials, thereby increasing competitiveness in the market, is certification or accreditation. Some programmes have academic requirements; others accept anyone who pays. Some are established by law; others are merely conferred by an association or group of practitioners who augment their own income by giving workshops and nepotistically supervising others. Like licensing, certification provides several advantages: it increases credibility, creates a critical mass for political lobbying, sometimes provides access to third-party payments and generally lends an enhanced marketability. Perusal of any urban phone directory provides examples such as: Certified Art Therapist and Certified Expressive Arts Therapist, Registered Clinical Counsellor, Registered Play Therapist, Certified Reality Therapist, Certified Master Rebirther, NLP Master Practitioner(TM), Master Hypnotist and Certified Hypnotherapist, Certified Traumatologist(TM), Certified Holotropic BreathWorker(TM), Certified Compassion Fatigue Specialist(TM), Certified EMDR Practitioner(TM) and Certified Master Time Line Therapy(TM) Practitioner.

A further means of establishing credibility is that of personal experience as a victim. Many people who choose to work with adult survivors of childhood trauma 'are coming to it from their own victimization' according to Marilyn Murray, a specialist in the field.[79] Ann Jones, author of *Next Time, She'll Be Dead*, supports such a view: 'I speak from experience. My father was a drunk, a wife beater, and a child abuser,'[80] as does Anne Wilson Schaef, in stating: 'my relationship addiction recovery process has been key in its interaction with my professional work and how I came to view my work.'[81]

Another way to compete effectively is to specialize or, as the APA terms it, 'finding the right niche in [the] new market.'[82] One fertile concept for creating marketplace niches is 'stress'. In 1945, Grinker and Spiegel reported on the reactions of Second World War combat fliers exposed to the threats and strain of battle, describing how the fliers were psychologically treated, outlining possible civilian applications.[83] Stress as a topic was picked up by postwar psychology and applied to a number of new areas, including 'life stress events' leading to physical illness,[84] 'executive stress' resulting in burnout,[85] and 'performance stress' causing academic failure or sexual dysfunction.[86] By the late 1980s a new array of specialists were emerging, who redefined stress as trauma. Using terms such as 'prisoner of childhood'[87] and 'inner child', they began to portray their patients as victims of trauma and treat them for the damage caused by events outside their control.

Psychologists received an enormous amount of publicity because of the claims of new techniques which often involved hypnosis and hypnoanalysis, regression therapy, NeuroLinguistic Programming™ or eye movement desensitization and reprogramming (EMDR). The mass media picked up the topic too. From talk shows to tabloids, these psychologists with their new specialities sold their wares as they described case after case in which individuals had uncovered their trauma and recovered. The subject matter contained sex and violence, qualities known to draw viewers, and the message was inspiring; success stories went unquestioned.[88]

A new field of specialization had been defined which offered practitioners a way to establish a business less affected by the tightening belt of the health-care industry. Thus began the Psychology Industry's current venture into manufacturing victims. Psychologists could now claim to be specialists in treating those who had been abused as children, or were victims of sexual abuse, of satanic abuse and so on. Psychologists' aggressive advertising began to show signs of the retooling that was going on within the Psychology Industry.

However, specialization may not be enough to compete successfully since many psychologists may end up claiming the same speciality. Creating a new one may be the solution; there will not be as many competitors, at least for a while. And to get the full benefit, the psychologist might consider claiming ownership of it as 'intellectual property' and registering it as a product with its own trademark. A number have done this with techniques they have developed (e.g. NLP, EMDR), thereby restricting others from using the speciality designation unless they obtain formal training sanctioned by the owner/psychologist. Those who are cunning enough to do this often ride the wave of their success to prestige and profit.

Ries and Trout describe inventing such a specialty as the Second Law of Marketing: 'The Law of Category.' 'If you can't be first in a category set up a new category you can be first in.'[89] Inventing a specialty usually means creating a new problem or treatment. In commercial manufacturing, most new products are a modification or an improvement of an existing product, or a new application of a current product. The same is true for most of the new specialities of the Psychology Industry. A variety of fields have opened up in this way, such as 'traumatology' and 'critical incidence stress (CIS) debriefing'. Once created, the next step is usually to establish an institute, society, foundation or centre to study and promote the area, followed by a book and lecture tour, a series of workshops and training programmes which then certify other psychologists, resulting in a hierarchy or pyramid of specialists.

The April 1995 bombing of the Federal Building in Oklahoma City provided an opportunity for 'traumatologists' to demonstrate their wares. In a programme called 'Operation Healing', they undertook to provide traumatology counselling. Some psychologists worked on-site in Oklahoma City while a nationwide free telephone number was set up that operated twenty-four hours a day. An organization called the Green Cross was created to 'support not just the Oklahoma Operation but others as well'. It was described as 'an organization that helps professionals in stricken areas help their neighbours grow healthy . . . As the Red Cross aids those in crisis, the Green Cross focuses on long-term struggles to recovery.' The organizers then determined that they needed to train others and that a 'curriculum' was needed 'that would enable them to do the work of healing the traumatized themselves'. A 'faculty' was assembled of volunteer psychologists from around the world, connected through the use of videos and the Internet. Four training workshops were scheduled, complete with a 'graduation ceremony' at which time registrants would receive their own credentials as registered traumatologists.[90]

Yvonne McEwan, a Scottish trauma expert, openly challenged this new specialty. In an invited address at the 1997 European Trauma Conference in London, she delivered the shocking message that professional counselling is largely a waste of time and does more to boost the ego of the counsellor than to help the victim. She declared the profession to be 'at best useless and at worst highly destructive to victims', and accused professional counsellors of 'creating a nation of victims in order to boost their flagging careers in the medical profession'. As McEwan sees it, 'the legal profession and medicine have colluded in the whole fabrication of people undergoing trauma' and 'by medicalising what is a non-medical condition and introducing therapy subject matter that is vastly abused, medicine is propping up a lot of dwindling careers.' This outspoken critic claims that 'the whole disaster scene has become a growth industry since the Bradford fire,' a fire at the local football grounds, in which more than forty fans died. In 1996 in Dunblane, Scotland, sixteen children aged four and five were killed along with their teacher by a man who then turned this gun on himself. McEwan points out that, in this case, 'there were far more counsellors than victims.'[91]

According to McEwan, many people, including some trauma counsellors, are nodding their heads in agreement.[92] However, despite her dismissive stance, the reactions to it, and people everywhere who shake their heads, quietly wondering about the merits of this 'coffee-cup therapy',[93] aggressive marketing strategies ensure that trauma counselling flourishes. The APA, for instance, has been lobbying federal, state and local governments for disaster-response plans and funding, stating that disaster victims need 'more long-term care'. Its demands include licensed clinicians to supervise, a strong research component to identify needs of people affected by the incident, and *mandatory* provision of mental-health services for rescue and relief workers.[94]

'The most powerful concept in marketing is owning a word in the prospect's mind,' and in the minds of many, 'trauma' has come to be a powerful psychological word. Consider the following recent examples:

- The 1996 flooding in Quebec lead to a relief programme which included the Red Cross paying for a maximum of twenty consultations for psychological assistance, up to $1,000 per evacuee. Similar services were offered to those involved in flooding in North Dakota and Manitoba in the spring of 1997.
- Trauma counsellors were rushed to Peggy's Cove, Nova Scotia on Canada's east coast after the 1998 crash of a Swissair jet killed all 220 on board. Rescue workers, family members, airline employees and residents all came to be viewed as victims. The Canadian military, which had assisted in search and clean-up, established a trauma programme specifically for its personnel.
- When a building being demolished in Canberra, Australia, exploded rather than imploded, resulting in injuries to spectators, a counselling service was set up within hours for the tens of thousands of tourists and locals who had come to watch the afternoon event.

These rescue missions are assumed to be necessary despite research which indicates that, with rare exceptions, psychological distress after disasters remits within a few weeks. Bickman, in a review of recent studies, states that 'disaster myths have been created by overemphasizing the relatively small increases in psychological distress following disasters across whole populations of survivors, or focusing on the small percentage of survivors whose lives are devastated by these events.'[95] Underscoring concepts of resilience, restoration of lost resources, re-establishment of social supports and a general return to normalcy, he stresses that priority should be placed on financial and social support, rather than interventions based on the mythology of trauma. Polak and his colleagues, in a controlled study of the effects of a sudden death of a family member, came to a similar conclusion that crisis intervention services were ineffective in reducing psychological consequences and that social factors are the important variables.[96]

A similar 'disaster-myth' entrepreneurial initiative is evident in critical incident stress debriefing (CISD), developed by Jeff Mitchell, a former volunteer firefighter and paramedic. He claims that a large proportion of emergency personnel experience some negative reaction to critical incidents. For many, he believes, these signs of stress, if left untreated, would 'develop into full-fledged post-traumatic stress disorders'. Consequently he designed CISD, a structured group intervention which focused on the identification and ventilation of emotions. The programme has become a burgeoning cottage industry of journals, books, workshops and lectures around the world.[97] Workshop registrants become trained CIS debriefers, a specialty used to gain contracts with emergency organizations, school boards, airlines and banks.

While CISD flourishes, progressively more critics, concerned about potential harm, are questioning the 'scientific evidence'. A battalion chief in a large metropolitan fire and rescue agency, writing about the ascendance of the CISD movement in his field, noted a comment made decades earlier by a hook and ladder captain: 'We used to have steel men and wooden wagons; now we have steel wagons and wooden men.'[98] He is one of an increasing number of people who are expressing concern that such procedures undermine the natural support and adaptation that keeps those with jobs like firefighting resilient. Adding support to this concern is the growing scientific literature which finds that the debriefing movement appears to have no appreciable preventive or palliative effect, and may, in fact, be responsible for an iatrogenic effect of causing the problems it claims to treat.[99]

Another, and one of the clearest examples of entrepreneurship, is John Gray's *Men Are from Mars, Women Are from Venus* concept. Since the release of his 1992 book, which sold 6 million copies, earning

Gray about $18 million, he has written five more with total sales of 9 million copies. He has also turned his concept into videotapes (3 million sold), audiotapes (1.3 million sold), audio CDs (130,000 shipped to date) and a board game. He markets seminars (at $35,000), workshops, Mars and Venus vacations, and hopes for a movie deal and a television sitcom.

As for counselling, Gray has a franchised line of Mars and Venus Counseling Centers operated by therapists who have paid $2,500 for training in the Mars and Venus 'technique', and pay a further $1,900, plus $300 per month royalties, for the rights to the name and logo.[100]

All of this on a PhD by correspondence and chutzpah.

'Cui bono?' – Who Is to Gain?

'For whose benefit are new services offered?' one might wonder. 'Is it the client and the community or the psychologist and the industry?'

Consider the Psychology Industry's recent intrusion into the developing medical area of reproductive technology: that of artificial insemination and embryo implantation. In a well-documented paper, Walker and Broderick show how psychologists are casting themselves as experts and judges in this bio-ethical field.[101] For instance, the creators of one screening programme believe that infertility has 'a deeper psychological meaning' and they approve potential parents accordingly. They write: 'we have found evidence of marked variations in [couples'] response to an unusual and potentially threatening predicament. Some appeared to have adapted well and could view this means to a child as entirely rational and psychologically acceptable. Others were more defensive and seemed reluctant to explore the deeper meaning of their infertility.'[102] On the basis of a single interview with a prospective couple, these psychologists in Solomonic style determine who deserves to be a parent and who does not.

They also instruct parents how they should act and warn them of what will happen if they don't do as instructed. They state that it is better: (1) for people undergoing treatment to talk to family, friends and counsellors about their use of donated gametes or embryos; (2) to tell a child of the method of conception and genetic background; and (3) for donors, recipients and children to know one another, regardless of circumstances or personal preferences for privacy. Failure to comply is interpreted as a pathological form of keeping secrets. They forecast that the refusal to inform others, including the child, of the use of 'donated material' will result in unhealthy family dynamics, impaired 'identity development' and 'genealogical bewilderment' in the children who will be 'driven to search for, and to seek reconciliation with, their biological ancestors'.[103]

Furthermore, the Psychology Industry identifies donors as potential clients by stressing the psychological effects of 'pre-natal adoption'. Referring to these individuals as the 'biological' fathers and mothers, they are told that they must consider 'the implications of another couple having your child' and of 'becoming a parent of children you may never know'.[104]

Every aspect of this potentially joyous experience becomes shrouded in a cloak of pathology. The eager parents are called 'substitute' or 'social' parents, and warned that 'donor insemination lends itself to secrecy in a way that adoption and assisted fertility techniques such as IVF cannot. This helps support the pretence that the conception, and therefore the family, is "normal".'[105] But according to psychologists, it isn't normal; it is, as Snowden and Mitchell term it, 'the artificial family'.[106] However, as Walker and Broderick write, 'perhaps the only ones who think that a child conceived through donor sperm belongs to an abnormal family are psychologists and social workers . . .'[107]

One can wonder how it is that such an esoteric medical area has become so quickly psychologized. Why is it easier to donate a kidney than an ovum, to receive someone else's heart than their sperm? The answer may be that the adoption business is diminishing and with it, the role that psychologists have carved for themselves within it, so that they must look for new sources of income. The growing business of assisted reproduction provides such an opportunity as the demand for it increases with the development and refinement of the technology. Current estimates are that as many as one couple in seven will have difficulty conceiving a child.[108] For the Psychology Industry, this represents a significant new market in which psychologists can posture as experts.

The intrusion of psychology into the domain of medicine is not new. In 1971, the APA president Kenneth Clark announced the 'era of psychotechnology', predicting the important role of psychoactive medications in the future of civilization. His ideas met with strong criticism from psychologists, not only because he proposed the drugging of 'all power-controlling world leaders' to 'assure their positive use of power and reduce or block the possibility of their using power destructively', but also because psychologists viewed themselves as opponents of psychiatric technology, having criticized psychiatrists for their use of drugs to treat symptoms and control people.

However, as the pendulum swings toward biological theories, psychologists have begun to express interest in prescribing privileges. Currently, they must refer their clients to psychiatrists or physicians for prescriptions and fear 'losing' them. One psychologist writes that he changed his mind on prescribing when one of his patients informed him that

> because she had to see her new psychiatrist for medication, she had decided to undertake her psychotherapy with this practitioner as well . . . If psychiatrists place a choke-hold on my patients' access to this therapy, I will devote my energy to gaining the right to provide, independently, the full range of mental health services. *Don't tread on me.*[109]

Psychoactive drugs are presenting a real threat to the Psychology Industry unless it can become involved in their prescription. For instance, psychologists have strongly argued that psychotherapy, specifically cognitive-behavioural therapy, is the treatment of choice for depression. But the development and growing popularity of Prozac and its derivatives (e.g. Zoloft), have made it a serious threat. In 1996, Prozac and Zoloft were prescribed to children and adolescents by US physicians more than 580,000 times, more than twice as often as in 1994 and almost ten times as often as in 1992, even though those drugs cannot be legally marketed for use by children. In 1996, worldwide sales of Prozac alone totalled US $2.3 billion.

The introduction in April 1998 of Viagra, the drug to overcome impotence and 'erectile dysfunction', has had a similar effect. In fact, early numbers suggested that this new wonder drug might even outsell Prozac. In its first two months, Viagra sold US$182 million worth of pills, outshining any other drug in history and becoming a threat to the sex-therapy industry. A Cleveland therapist states: 'Viagra is a threat to sex therapy precisely because it is a drug designed to take our "best customer".' So the Psychology Industry must push even harder to gain prescription privileges.

Although the proposal for prescribing privileges initially met with hesitation, by 1996 the APA's board of directors had approved model legislation for prescriptive authority, and allocated funds to support efforts to lobby for state-level prescription privileges for practitioners.[110] The profession that once declared itself as the alternative to psychiatry is now trying to turn itself into a pseudo-psychiatry, blurring the age-old distinction between medicine and psychology and provoking a turf war.

Proponents of the scheme argue that the right to prescribe will increase the likelihood that drugs 'are appropriately utilized, if used at all, and will ensure that practitioners can address society's pressing needs . . . in a safe, cost-effective and competent manner'.[111] But why would these expectations be realistic? As DeNelsky points out, 'there is a powerful seductiveness about medications.'[112] Drugs are easily provided, offer a quick fix and give the practitioner a sense of power. Already concerns exist that drugs are being overused and, with an increased number of minimally trained prescribers, it is difficult to imagine that this would not escalate. Aided by the forceful push of the pharmaceutical companies which provide large amounts of funding for research, education and travel to conferences supported by them, there is a strong likelihood that psychologists would do more and more prescribing. It is equally conceivable that this seductiveness may lure them beyond current prescribing practices into the use of drugs to create a happier society free of worry and sadness and their mandatory use to control violent, aggressive, sexual or addictive behaviours deemed unacceptable by society. Already one psychologist, James Goodwin, has gained international attention for his promotion of Prozac as the treatment of choice for complaints of violence, low self-esteem, chronic irritability, eating problems, hypersexuality and so on. 'I have this fantasy of pouring [Prozac] in the water,' he has stated. 'If I put out a good product and people are healthier and happier, that's fine by me. I don't mind being Dr Feelgood.'[113]

Although Goodwin may be at the extreme, he exemplifies the profession's dissatisfaction with its current status and its desire to expand its market and its power.

And the Beat Goes On

> *An influential group of therapists is promoting a new scare: children who molest other children. Those who question the murky evidence are said to be in denial. But it is the kids, taken from home and given intense therapy, who might be suffering the most.*[114]

The Psychology Industry's induced public hysteria about sexual abuse is creating yet another new specialization: 'children who molest'.

Coined by the psychologist Toni Cavanaugh Johnson in 1988, this diagnostic description has been applied to children as young as two, for 'inappropriate' behaviours such as diddling, licking, flashing, mooning, masturbating compulsively, looking up under girls' skirts, lying on top of a girl in bed; even using sexual language or asking endless questions about sex. This has led to siblings, cousins and playmates being diagnosed with 'sexual behaviour problems', charged with assault and removed from their families. And members of the Psychology Industry are seeking the inclusion of 'juvenile sex offending' into the *DSM*, the catalogue of psychopathologies.

In the early 1990s, the journalist Mark Sauer watched as Johnson and a social worker, Kee MacFarlane, presented their ideas at a professional conference. He was astonished. 'First they state that there is no research – that we really don't know anything about normal children's sexual behaviour,' he recalls. 'Then out come the pie charts and graphs and they go on for an hour defining this new abnormality. And everybody is madly taking notes.'

Sauer had reason to be suspicious of MacFarlane and the clinic she worked for, the Children's Institute International (CII) in Los Angeles. His newspaper had published some of the only sceptical coverage of the 1980s McMartin Preschool satanic ritual abuse trials. MacFarlane had headed the team that interrogated nearly 400 children for the prosecution and found 369 to have been victimized in bizarre rituals. Except for one, none of the children mentioned abuse until they got to CII. After the jury saw MacFarlane's taped interviews, full of leading, hectoring questions, they voted to acquit the defendants.[115]

Johnson and MacFarlane are not alone in promoting this new specialization. By the mid-1990s, the Vermont-based Safer Society Foundation database listed 50 residential and 396 nonresidential programmes that treat 'sex offenders' under twelve. In addition, two studies that provided therapy and evaluated the best treatment approach for hundreds of 'sexualized' children under twelve in the states of Vermont, Oklahoma and Washington were funded at a cost of $1 million. And 'at the 1995 Association for the Treatment of Sex Abusers conference, about 80 percent of the exhibition tables featured literature on such programs for children and adolescents.'

Such programmes have already become part of the Psychology Industry, with 'children's group work' and 'steps for recovery'. For instance, David McWhirter, a social worker and one of the United States' most prominent therapists of juvenile offenders, is quoted as saying about one twelve-year-old: 'the boy didn't want to confess guilt, the first stage required for "recovery".' Barbara Bonner, chief researcher of one of the million-dollar studies, admits that such processes are 'value driven' and based on what the psychologists 'consider to be appropriate and in the best interest of children'. She continues: 'We will probably never know the harm [of children behaving sexually] . . . we don't have long term outcomes. They [the children] may turn out to be normal.'

Despite Bonner's concessions and the concerns expressed by others, psychologists have gone about establishing for themselves this new specialization, leading Judith Levine to comment:

> with little supportive evidence, the new children-who-molest experts have persuaded the child protective systems they work for that 'sex-offense-specific' therapy is necessary for any kid with a 'sexual behaviour problem.' They insist this therapy, whose methodologies derive from their own theories, can be practised only by them or others they have trained.[116]

'This all reminds me of heroic gynecology (during the early twentieth century), which regarded the birth process itself as a pathological thing,' says Vern Bullough, distinguished professor emeritus at SUNY and author or editor of over fifty books on sexuality. 'What we've got now is heroic intervention in childhood sexuality by people who don't know what they are talking about.'[117]

Something for Nothing

While the development and promotion of specialities are of direct benefit to those who claim specialist status, they also have a pay-off to the Psychology Industry as a whole, as they serve to further psychologize the human experience. A release from APA describing its 'Disaster Response Network' (DRN) exposes the pathologizing and promotional aspects:

> The California fires and earthquake. The Midwest floods. Hurricanes Andrew and Iniki. The shooting on the Long Island commuter train and the World Trade Center bombing. These disasters have had a devastating impact on the lives of thousands

> of Americans. Their losses are, many times, unfathomable: homes, communities, jobs and sometimes, loved ones. As individuals and communities begin to pick up the pieces of their lives, they often times neglect the need for mental health care, something that disaster survivors desperately need at a time when they can least afford it financially. *If left untreated, these needs can develop into chronic problems that are disabling to people in both their professional and personal lives* . . . The mental health needs of the national disasters have been monumental . . . In addition to the short-term crisis intervention services the DRN offers survivors, the network *helps them to identify local resources for ongoing psychological assistance.*[118]

While this sounds altruistic, especially when described as 'APA's centennial gift to the nation', a look at documents on 'Diversifying Your Sources of Practice Income' suggests an ulterior motive: 'Providing public sector services on a pro bono basis is *an effective marketing tool* that may create other professional opportunities involving compensation.'[119] Perhaps it is with this in mind that most psychologists provide such pro bono services.[120]

The move towards specialization has spawned a number of new subindustries. There are now specialists in the treatment of post-traumatic stress disorder in people whose friends and acquaintances have committed suicide, people who have lost a pet, who were fired from their job, who experienced a divorce or death, who are veterans of the Second World War and experiencing memories due to the fiftieth anniversary, or who have experienced gender discrimination.[121] Similarly, there are specialists in the addiction and recovery of those dependent on and thereby victims of love, sex, 'urgency', religion, shopping, on-line computing, food, prostitution and so on.[122]

The invention of a specialty would seem to be restricted only by the limits of one's imagination, as the following illustrate:

- 'Licensed Volunteer Therapy Dog'. This designation is awarded to animals who complete a series of special obedience courses and pass a test at one of the thirty-five US chapters of Therapy Dogs International.[123]

- Llama therapy. Llamas are being used to 'teach teenage offenders to develop affection and concern for other creatures' and in the treatment of abused children. In British Columbia, the Llama Therapeutic Group offers stress management.[124]
- Compassion fatigue. The occupational hazard of psychologists who suffer from the excessive emotional demands of their clients and the negative effects of working with traumatized or troubled clients.[125] The Traumatology Institute offers a powerful Accelerated Recovery Program culminating in certification as Compassion Fatigue Specialists.[126]
- Legal abuse syndrome. This 'can strike crime victims, witnesses, litigants, attorneys – anyone who has dealt with the American system of laws and courts.'[127]
- 'Enslavement by e-mail'. A report on research conducted by a coalition of Canadian mental-health organizations announces that the onslaught of e-mail and the explosion of other new technologies can make workers psychologically and mentally ill.[128]

Once the issues of credibility and product line are resolved, the next and all-important issue facing psychologists is publicity. Consider the following advertised services:

- 'The Psychology Network Introduces Live Conversations with Psychologists 24 Hours a Day, 7 Days a Week, from Any Telephone.' 'If you are concerned by an issue in the middle of the night, you don't have to wait for counselling, there's always a doctor waiting to talk with you, instead of the other way around,' said Rich Ralston, vice president of marketing for the Psychology Network, Inc.[129]
- Internet services such as:

  – On-line training in various psychotherapy techniques such as cognitive therapy, in which 'the program covers all of the basic features of cognitive therapy, and offers a "hands-on" experience in using common treatment procedures.'[130]

– CyberAnalysis, a source of one-to-one psychotherapy, offered by a British psychiatrist. Dr Razzaque's therapy typically involves one preliminary session, followed by more intensive sessions booked in groups of four and punctuated by strategic e-mails containing specific analytical tools and perspectives.[131]

- The Recovery Network, a television channel with programming exclusively on topics 'from alcohol to drugs, to depression, sex, obsession, eating disorders, family violence, compulsive gambling and sexual abuse'. An article in the *New Republic* described this network as 'the end of the line, the logical terminus for a culture in love with its own dysfunction . . . a "round-the-clock" media showcase of addiction and anomie . . . [a] proudly pathological cable channel . . .'[132]

Until recently, psychologists, social workers and psychiatrists were prohibited from advertising. Their argument that this gave unlicensed psychologists an unfair advantage was supported by the Bureau of Competition of the US Federal Trade Commission, making way for broad market-driven advertising. Although phrased by licensing bodies and professional associations in term of complying with federal regulations, the unacknowledged benefit of this change was to increase the visibility of the Psychology Industry. Now psychologists show little caution regarding media interviews or talk shows and freely extol their services, making exorbitant claims about what users can expect, even if their claims contradict research findings.

Noble Lying

Are the extravagant claims and advertisements of the Psychology Industry merely false expectations, or do they constitute deception and fraud?

According to Kottler:

> Telling clients that we can help them is assuredly helpful even if it is not strictly true . . . We would lose clients very quickly if after every bungled interpretation . . . we muttered 'Oops, I blew that one.' *We would never get a client to come back if we were completely honest with them* . . . the client may need to believe in this lie . . .[133]

Some forms of deception have always been a part of psychological practice. When confronted by moral objections to therapists deceiving their patients, a contemporary of Freud's, Pierre Janet, responded:

> I am sorry that I cannot share these exalted and beautiful scruples . . . My belief is that the patient wants a doctor who will cure; that the doctor's professional duty is to give any remedy that will be useful, and to prescribe it in the way in which it will do most good. Now I think that bread pills are medically indicated in certain cases and that they will act far more powerfully if I deck them out with impressive names. When I prescribe such a formidable placebo, I believe that I am fulfilling my professional duty.[134]

Janet's (and Kottler's) assumption was that patients want and need to be treated as children by paternal and protective, if not always honest, psychologists, and that it is in the best interest of these patients to lie, for 'there are some to whom, as a matter of strict moral obligation, we must lie'.

Thus deception has become a cornerstone of the Psychology Industry.[135] Kottler writes: 'If lying to a client, deliberately or unintentionally, is unethical since it promotes deceit and deception, perhaps it is just as unethical to be *completely truthful.*'[136] Whether it is expressed in terms of creating positive expectations which are believed to be essential for a good therapy outcome, or fostering unconditional acceptance and positive regard, or giving unquestioning support to a claim of abuse, the Noble Lie has gained acceptance in the Psychology Industry.

A psychologist, when asked about the 'facts' he had presented in his bestseller dealing with a case of satanic abuse, replied that it didn't really matter 'whether or not they were technically true, that was immaterial'; he didn't want to 'nit-pick about facts'.[137] For these and many other psychologists, it doesn't matter whether facts are true or whether what they say is honest; what matters is that clients believe them.[138]

Recently, Alan Scheflin, a law professor, went beyond acknowledging the deception. In addressing a conference on hypnosis and psychotherapy, he encouraged psychologists to consider the ethical responsibility to intentionally deceive their clients:

> The point I want to make is the assumption that implanting false memories is wrong. I would like to raise the issue of whether we are right to say it is wrong . . . When we get through the false memory issue perhaps we can start to debate the serious question . . . that *therapists are in fact social influence purveyors* and it is your job to use those techniques. And hypnosis will lead the way into the social influence literature. And then we can start to talk about *the ethics of using false memories therapeutically*.[139]

Thus, to Scheflin and the audience which gave him a standing ovation, the end justifies the means even if the means is to mislead, deceive and lie to patients, and to create a false history of their lives.

Perhaps another reason that Scheflin got such a rousing round of applause on that occasion was that he was promising psychologists that soon 'there will be a point – though there has not been one yet' when they would find the power that 'would make therapists more effective in treating the problems of the patient'.[140] His message was encouraging to the many psychologists who carry on their daily practice of professional deception, creating an image of themselves as confident and self-assured while inwardly feeling anxious and inept.

A study of 421 psychologists revealed that psychologists wish to be seen as 'irrepressibly superior'; as dependable, capable, conscientious, intelligent, friendly, honest, adaptable, responsible, reasonable and considerate.[141] Deceptive image-making is seen as essential for success.

Arons and Spiegel, in a chapter subtitled 'The Wizard of OZ Exposed', wrote: 'When we [psychologists] sit in our consultation rooms, we often try to present *a carefully sculpted image* to our patients . . . At times, we are much like the Wizard of OZ, trying to make an impressive presentation while hoping that the curtain we hide behind won't be pulled aside to reveal more vulnerable parts of ourselves.'[142] And one female therapist added: 'My clients aren't particularly open-minded. I fear their rejection. Many wouldn't like me if they really knew me, and that wouldn't be very good for my practice.'[143]

The Psychology Industry's solution to this dilemma is to hide any insecurities or inadequacies. Now this wouldn't necessarily be bad, for after all it is a strategy adopted in many businesses, if it were not for two difficulties: it makes it difficult for psychologists to be human and to admit 'I don't know', and it fosters a 'one-up' relationship between psychologists and their clients.

For some yet unexplained reason, a majority of the public is gullible to this deception. It is inclined to believe what psychologists say on television, on the radio, in books or in sessions. Perhaps it is, as David Smail says, that even though 'all promises that we may return to the blissful ease of infancy are false . . . wishful dreaming renders one vulnerable to commercial promises of its coming true . . .'[144] Perhaps it is the cultural pressures of Western society to accord an honorific status to professionals, particularly if they can parade as scientists and experts. Whatever the reason, the psychologist maintains the status of an 'acknowledged expert'. And reaps the benefits.

Kottler, writing *On Being a Therapist*, candidly said:

> In exchange for spending forty-five minutes listening to someone talk and telling them what we think about what they said, we receive enough money to buy ten books or a whole night on vacation. It is absurd. It would almost seem that even with the hardships of being a therapist, *we have a good thing going.*[145]

5

The Technology of Victim-Making

Psychotherapy is a service, a business, an industry, yet the mystique of psychotherapy endures beyond all reason. As a profit-making industry, psychotherapy wants an informed customer.

Robert Langs

If psychologists have a good thing going, then they have an even better thing going when they simplify their thinking and streamline their treatments. With the goals of the Psychology Industry being to broaden the market, increase sales and raise income, there has been a trend towards mechanization. For this, an informed customer is not what the Psychology Industry wants. Instead, it directs its advertising to those who, having a 'psychologically-prone personality', are amenable to simplistic thinking and authoritarian assembly-line techniques.

The 'Psychologically-Prone' Personality

Millions of people are exposed to psychological influence each year. Not all succumb. Some have little inclination to the procedures; some resist the pressures; some detect the coercive nature and quit. By no means do all become its willing victims. Those who do seem to be characterized by a 'psychologically-prone personality':

- Seeing the world in terms of psychological notions.
- Being emotionally preoccupied and reactive.
- Being predisposed to imagination and fantasy.
- Being open to psychological suggestion and influence.
- Seeking direction and guidance in living.
- Wanting simple solutions and answers.
- Attributing authority to those they view as experts.

They uphold what Thomas Wolfe refers to as 'the new alchemical dream'. Whereas 'the old alchemical dream was changing base metal into gold . . . the new alchemical dream is changing one's personality – remaking, remodeling, elevating and polishing one's very self . . . observing, studying and doting on it.'[1] As the ancient alchemists were inducted into secret societies and magical orders, those with a psychologically-prone personality are inducted into the psychological society.

Probably their most salient feature is suggestibility. They are easily seduced by the rhetoric of psychology; influenced by the subtle communication of experts and easily persuaded by the directive guidance offered in psychotherapy. As Hans Strupp observed: 'all forms of psychotherapy employ suggestion . . . the patient's suitability for psychotherapy is based on his potential openness to suggestion.'[2]

The role of suggestion can be found throughout history: from the sleep temples of the ancient Egyptians to the 'magnetic cures' of Mesmer, the early work of Freud and the effects of medical placebos. It is apparent in the fear-appeal claims of the expert, in the artful influences of the psychotherapist, and in the deliberate suggestions of the hypnotist.

Psychologically-prone individuals are vulnerable to experts who, in lectures, workshops and writings, identify themes in society, address them in vivid psychological terms and suggest solutions which seem effortlessly achievable. For instance, Slaby in writing about 'aftershock,' which he defines as a 'delayed effect of trauma, crisis and loss', vividly introduces the topic by saying that 'once, almost everyone assumed that aftershock was exclusively contracted during war . . . But these are the larger-than-life examples, the terrifying horror stories that are the rare exceptions to the rule . . .' He continues by generalizing trauma to include all sorts of upsets and unpleasant feelings, to which anyone can relate: '*We all* suffer from aftershock, maybe less violently but still at a price we shouldn't have to pay. In fact, aftershock is the disease of today.'[3] And he optimistically concludes:

> Together, we have seen the ways to avoid aftershock and the stress that always joins it. What is left?
> Only this: a message for the future, for a world where we can live up to our full potential without fear, without anxiety, without the past to haunt our days . . .
> Welcome, then, with me, crisis. We may never conquer death, but we can conquer life and make it the best it can be.
> Together we can stop aftershock for good.
> Welcome to a brave – and exciting – new world.[4]

In reading this, the psychologically-prone person can imagine the horror (and aftershock) of war, and then slide the slippery slope into accepting the suggestion of personal aftershock which Slaby says 'we all' experience, and end up believing in the psychological promise of a utopian ('brave, new') world.

Two additional means of suggestive influence exist for those already in psychological treatment: one subtle and almost imperceptible, and the other, directive and hypnotic-like.

Psychologically-prone clients, believing that the therapist has specialized knowledge, often search their psychologists' behaviour, moods and remarks for hidden cues, which will influence their thinking and actions. Even the slightest reaction or response can have a great influence. As Frank notes: 'The very subtlety and unobtrusiveness of the therapist's influencing maneuvers, coupled with his explicit disclaimer that [the psychologist] is exerting any influence, may increase his influencing power.'[5] Functioning as 'indirect suggestions', these forms of suasion have power over a large number of users, heightening their responsiveness to therapy and extending the influence of psychologists.

Evidence of such subtle influence is available from numerous sources. People in Freudian analysis have been shown to produce Freudian dreams, while those in Jungian therapy have jungian dreams, an effect which Calestro explains as follows: 'the underlying mechanism apparently involves a process of suggestion in which the patient responds to overt or covert suggestions by the therapists that certain phenomena will occur.'[6] Others have demonstrated the ability of therapists to influence the values of their patients to come in line with their own. Welkowitz and his colleagues arbitrarily assigned clients to therapists and subsequently found that the values of the therapists resembled those of their own patients more than those seen by other therapists, and that the similarity of values tended to increase over time or length of treatment.[7] Similarly, a study by Rosenthal found a positive relationship between ratings of improvement and the change of clients' moral values towards those of the psychologists, *with respect to sex, aggression and authority.*[8] Since such moral conversion is possible, it is no wonder that psychologists with a victim-oriented philosophy can intentionally or inadvertently manufacture victims.

The study of hypnosis has much to contribute to the understanding of the psychologically-prone personality, which is susceptible not only to the indirect cues inherent in psychological treatment, but also to the hypnotic-like suggestions of psychologists. For instance, Lynn and Rhue suggest that 'imaginative involvement', an aspect of hypnosis, plays a defensive function for abused children in that traumatized children can construct a world of fantasy into which they can retreat as an 'adaptive means of coping with negative environmental factors'.[9] They theorize that this fantasy-proneness then extends into adult life as an effect of the early trauma. However, the connection between reported childhood trauma and imaginative involvement of hypnosis is correlational; so it is just as likely that the psychologically-prone person's susceptibility to therapist influence results in client characteristics similar to those of the disorder, an iatrogenic effect, as it is that the disorder causes one to be hypnotically responsive. Consider the following suggestive instructions given by a psychologist to those who have not yet remembered being sexually abused: 'If you sense that you were sexually abused and have no memories of it, it's likely that you were . . . Spend time *imagining* that you were sexually abused, without worrying about accuracy or having your ideas make sense . . . When you feel ready, ask yourself . . . Who would have been likely perpetrators?'[10]

Individuals with a psychologically-prone personality are more apt to be open to such suggestions, whether or not abuse ever occurred, since fantasy-prone individuals are particularly susceptible to distortions in their memory.[11] Bryant reports a study intended to investigate the relationship between fantasy-proneness and the age at which reported childhood sexual abuse occurred.[12] The subjects, women who had reported sexual abuse in childhood, were assessed for their tendency to become imaginatively involved in internal events, and the extent to which fantasy played a role in their adult functioning. Bryant not only confirmed a correlational relationship between fantasy-proneness and reports of childhood abuse, he also found that 'reports of abuse at a younger age are associated with higher levels of fantasy proneness'. This finding could lead many to conclude that trauma plays 'a causal role in the development of fantasy-based modes of coping'. However, the reverse is equally plausible; that these women, who were all more hypnotizable and prone to fantasy than those in the control group, are more likely to use their imagination to construct memories (pseudomemories) of abusive events at an early age. It is worth noting that the subjects in this study were all involved in an imagery-based treatment programme and that the abuse they reported was only assumed to be true.

In discussing the possibility that the diagnosis and stories of Sybil, the celebrated case of Multiple Personality Disorder (MPD) that gained public attention from the book and subsequent film of the same name, were the product of the therapist, Herbert Spiegel says:

> that is one of the biggest difficulties with working with the concept of causation in psychotherapy. It is the grand illusion that we have

> inherited from Freud. Freud's concept was that you had to get to the truth, and unless you get the truth no therapeutic effect can take place. So, in the pursuit of the truth we become engaged in story telling and we impose our hypothesis on the patient by the way we ask our questions. Highly suggestible (psychologically-prone) people will of course respond in a way that can please the doctors, especially if there is a good rapport between them.

And he continues by describing a victim-making process consistent with that of synthetic and counterfeit-victims:

> These patients are full of anger and guile. They feel victimized and tend to blame others for their misbehavior. They then find a doctor who can conjoin with them to develop a story of abuse which appears to be a multiple personality disorder, thus giving them a new kind of status in society. They will make use of all this alleged or real abuse which took place in their life, as a way of getting recognition: 'Look, I'm a multiple!' They don't have to do it on their own anymore. Nowadays, they have the collusion of a therapist who is showing them how to do it. And then they can have hospital stays for months to years that the insurance companies pay for.[13]

Designing Simplistic Theories

> *Oh, don't take that too seriously. That's something I dreamed up on a rainy Sunday afternoon.*
>
> Freud's response to a question about the logic of a particular psychoanalytic theorem.[14]

The two key components of any manufacturing industry are design and production. In the Psychology Industry, 'design' involves the construction of theories which supposedly unravel the mysteries of life, making them understandable and curable.

In a society in which truth is most often determined by popular opinion and in which justice is a product of legal machinations, the profession of psychology might have been an oasis of intellectual freedom. But psychology surrendered this privilege, becoming preoccupied with business issues of growth and profit. While psychologists have focused on making their reputations and their fortunes, the Psychology Industry has become a conceptual warehouse of junk science, full of harmful ideas and malicious influences.[15] It has chosen to create theories for popular use rather than theories based on research, often reducing them to simplistic concepts out of which come marketable services rather than further investigation and greater understanding.

In examining the 'American mind', Allan Bloom observed that the 'search for material causes and reduction of higher or more complex phenomena to lower or simpler ones are generally accepted procedures'.[16] Nowhere is this more evident than in the Psychology Industry, where ideas and discoveries are quickly metamorphosed into pop concepts and fad therapies.

'Life stress events' is a case in point. In 1967, Holmes and Rahe, in an effort to quantify the effect of recent life changes on physical health, created a list of forty-three events, the Social Readjustment Rating Scale of Recent Experiences (SRE).[17] The list contained changes that were both positive (e.g. job promotion and marriage) and negative (e.g. divorce and arrest). Each was given a Life Change Unit (LCU) determined by having diverse groups of subjects rate the amount of readjustment required, from 1 to 100 units. Subjects then responded to each item by indicating whether they had experienced that event during the past two years. The researchers showed that life events cluster significantly in a two-year period prior to the onset of an illness. As a research scale, the SRE was interesting. It initiated a whole field of research into the effects of life changes. The scale was altered, refined and criticized; the theory was applauded, questioned and attacked.[18]

However, many psychologists, only superficially aware of the ongoing debate and subsequent refinements, grabbed the SRE, which was never meant to be used as a clinical tool, and began to use it in their work. Executives fired from their jobs were being given the scale as part of their relocation package. Medical patients were completing it to 'help them understand the psychological aspects of their disease or illness'. And psychotherapy patients were routinely filling it in as part of the battery of psychological tests before treatment. In some cases, it was being used to predict or explain physical illness. But in the majority of cases, it was being misused as a scale to measure overall stress which could then be related to any or all behaviours of the clients. Recent events became the explanation whereby people became labelled as victims of stress.

Despite the constructive controversy among the researchers, and in spite of the revisions and changes being made to both the scale and the concept, the Psychology Industry persisted in its misuse of the scale. As one psychologist commented, 'the scale is easy to give and score, and it's interesting to patients. It doesn't matter whether it is reliable or not, it's simple and it gives us something to talk about.'

But not only was stress something to talk about, the Psychology Industry argued that it was something to be treated. Health psychology was created out of the notion that if stress could lead to illness, then eliminating it could lead to 'wellness'. While this possibility could be applied to everything from arthritis to colitis to dermatitis, two areas drew most of the attention: heart attacks and cancer.

In the late 1950s, two American cardiologists, Friedman and Rosenman, provided an explanation of coronary illness that hit the jackpot: 'we feel that a complex of emotional reactions which we categorize as Type A behavior is *the principal cause* of coronary illness.'[19] Type A behaviour was characterized by time urgency, explosive speech, and extremes in impatience, competitiveness, job involvement and achievement striving.

Their findings showed a strong association between Type A behaviour and coronary disease.[20] Was it cause or correlation? The Psychology Industry preferred to consider it as cause, following a form of reasoning which Plous and Piattelli-Palmarini have called 'illusory correlation';[21] erroneously assuming that a characteristic or symptom is proof of cause.[22]

Based on the assumption that Type A behaviour caused heart attacks, the Psychology Industry began to teach stress-reduction strategies and to use behaviour modification to change Type A behaviours. They ignored later research which, by the end of the 1980s, was entirely unsupportive of their technology.[23] The psychological treatment of cardiovascular disease illustrates a point that Parloff once made: 'No form of psychotherapy has ever been initiated without a claim that it has unique therapeutic advantages, and no form of psychotherapy has ever been abandoned because of its failure to live up to these claims.'[24]

Another illustration comes from the research into the unavoidable life event of dying, which provides the basis for another enduring psychological technology. In 1981, Kubler-Ross's study of terminally ill patients led her to identify five psychological stages involved in preparing to die: denial, anger, bargaining, depression, and acceptance.[25]

She described these as usual stages, acknowledging that not everyone would go through them or necessarily experience them in this order. However, the Psychology Industry has taken possession of this model, simplifying, altering and applying it to fit different target groups. Describing the steps as psychological necessities, it has created a constricted technology, a procedure for 'psychologically healthy dying', while simultaneously creating an industry that ensures that this constriction will endure; that of bereavement counselling, 'grief work' and palliative care.

But, as with the life stress events work, the research evaluating the model presents a very different and more complex picture, exposing a number of myths. When people who have suffered major traumas are studied, almost half seem not to experience intense anxiety, depression or grief after the loss.[26] And over the years, the roll-with-the-punches people are found to remain well adjusted and healthy. Pennebaker, critical of this simplistic approach, says: 'Not everyone progresses through stages in grieving or coping. In fact, as many as half of all adults may face torture, divorce, the loss of a loved one, or other catastrophe and not exhibit any major sign of depression or anxiety. By definition, then, a substantial number of people may not benefit from attempts to influence their coping strategies.'[27]

Another researcher, George Bonanno, offers his empirical analysis of the so-called grief-work hypothesis: the widely held assumption that venting negative emotions and 'telling your story' are necessary for regaining mental health. So far, his experiments have yielded intriguingly counterintuitive results, suggesting that grief-stricken people who express intense negative emotions when discussing their loss appear to do worse in the long term, than those that keep it in.

Bonanno is not alone in drawing these conclusions. Wortman and Silver conclude that there is little evidence that 'those who initially show minimal distress following loss are likely to become significantly depressed at a later point'. And the Dutch researchers Margaret and Wolfgang Stroebe state: 'In our view, bereavement is an issue that needs to be understood from a sound base of theoretically oriented and empirically derived knowledge and not purely on subjective, descriptive accounts.'[28]

These findings come at a time when the 'bereavement industry', as Bonanno calls it, is flourishing and those in the business are not easily influenced by them. The Association of Death Education and Counselling boasts more than 2,000 members. At its 1997 annual meeting, where Bonanno presented his findings, 'attendees enjoyed "complimentary massages" in one of the conference rooms or visited an odd mourning mini-mall offering books like *Why Are the Casseroles Always Tuna? A Loving Look at the Lighter Side of Grief*, while they shared their own painful stories and talked of "caring" and "love".'[29]

Where once Kubler-Ross's model gave a glimpse into the unfathomable experience of one's own imminent death and a means by which others might understand the vacillations in the moods and thinking of those approaching death, it has now been generalized so that the stages apply not only to the dying one but to the survivor of the death of a parent, of a child, of a spouse or a friend, even of a poodle or parakeet. A book by Quackenbush, for example, describes how he 'thoughtfully examines the full range of normal emotions (depression, guilt, denial, and anger)' for grieving pet owners.[30] Other psychologists have applied the model to a variety of situations in which the word 'loss' can be loosely applied: 'loss of a job', 'loss of an object' (such as in a burglary) or 'loss of a friendship' (as in relocating because of work). A theoretical concept, useful to the study of thanatology, has become, like addiction, post-traumatic shock disorder and many other psychological concepts, an industrial mould to be applied willy-nilly to a whole array of identified issues.

Psychological Nostrums

> *Are the emotionally distressed the recipients of the fruits of a true psychological revolution or the victims of a cheap psychic nostrum?*
>
> Martin Gross

From the witches' brews of ancient times to the travelling medicine shows, from copper bracelets to Kickapoo Indian oil, society has always had an abundance of secret concoctions and panaceas to cure its ailments. People have been gullible to promises of easy ways to gain hair or lose weight, so it is hardly surprising that they are open to easy solutions even for personal and interpersonal discomforts, which less affluent societies would regard as trivial. In the first half of this century, one of the most successful psychic nostrums was Couéism. Known otherwise as autosuggestion, it combined some of the rationale of the modern Psychology Industry with the rituals of ancient times. Emile Coué, a French pharmacist and a student of hypnosis, instructed persons suffering from nervous disorders to tell themselves repeatedly throughout the day: 'Every day and in every way I am getting better and better.' For a few decades, his popularity and influence were phenomenal.[31]

Belief in something simple is the sign of a nostrum, whether it is a magic potion, a miracle tonic or a psychological formula. Psychological cure-alls did not begin nor did they end with Coué's invention. Some years ago Bergin and Garfield said:

> it is a matter of concern that so many new therapies that have no empirical support are invented and introduced by licensed practitioners, but even more so by entrepreneurial unlicensed persons. Numerous treatments are also applied by people who have merely attended a workshop or two in a procedure and then considered themselves to be experts. It is also unfortunate that fads continue to dot the landscape of the mental health professionals and that a fair amount of magical thinking regarding the power to change people is associated with such movements.[32]

Whether they are psychic nostrums, therapy movements or treatment fads, the technologies of the Psychology Industry have a common theme: 'You have to get worse before you get better!'

The addiction technologies and the trauma/abuse technologies share a four-stage model of manufacturing victims. They begin with people who have bad feelings or behaviours, and then cause them to feel worse as they begin to identify themselves as victims. Once the identity is established, they start the recovery process with the ultimate goal or promise of a new life and a new identity. The whole process can be considered a technology because it treats all victims identically, putting them through the same procedures.

FIGURE 1

Four Stage Technology

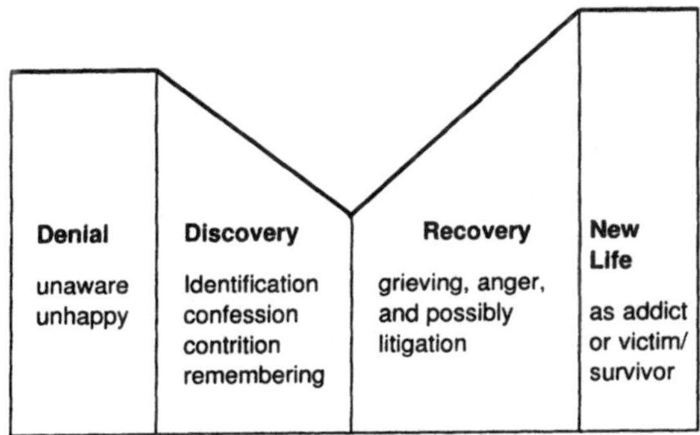

Addictions

Despite the current attention to trauma, the addiction industry remains the most profitable victim-making enterprise. Twenty-five million Americans are considered to be alcoholics. When those addicted to drugs and a range of behaviours are included and expanded to encompass their families, friends and associates, the number soars to 250 million, a number close to the population of North America. As Stanton Peele states, the addiction movement has produced 'the multimillion dollar alcohol-as-a-disease treatment industry and now a host of new diseases, such as being the child-of-a-person-with-the-disease-of-alcoholism'.[33]

It began with the treatment of heroin addicts but really came into its own with Alcoholics Anonymous (AA) and the myriad of off-shoots. AA started as a private fellowship based on the proposition that alcoholics are able to achieve sobriety only with the ongoing support of God and other alcoholics. The movement was gradually co-opted by medicine and psychology, resulting in a hybrid theory of addiction as both a bad behaviour and a disease. In 1985, Holden wrote in *Science* describing alcoholism as 'the neglected disease in medical education' and stating that 'alcoholism, as a chronic disease, offers "a fantastic vehicle to teach other concepts"'.[34] What Holden didn't say was that 'with the attribution of disease, the individual is delivered up to a body of institutional experts – psychiatrists, child guidance counsellors, physicians, alcohol treatment practitioners, social workers – who seek the person's rehabilitation. In becoming technical objects, the deviants give rise to a new group of control agents and agencies whose power is suspect.'[35]

The Psychology Industry had already recognized alcoholism as a prototype and had begun taking cuttings from the stem, creating variations of addiction as a disease of helplessness to be identified and treated by addiction specialists. Psychologists chose to endorse medicine's disease model, allowing technologies to be developed and applied. By adopting this notion of addictions as diseases and those addicted as victims, the Psychology Industry encouraged people to believe that the problem is not of their own making, thus excusing the behaviour, increasing the readiness to accept the diagnosis, and sanctioning forced treatment as an alternative to incarceration or job loss.

The growth in addiction treatments has involved casting a wider net to catch more varieties of addictions and persuading the public of the progressive nature of these 'diseases'. From psychologists and profit-making treatment centres, the message goes out: if you think you have a drinking problem, then indeed you do; or if parents suspect a child of smoking marijuana, this 'is probably only the tip of the iceberg' and they should make any financial sacrifice necessary to ensure that the child gets treatment for 'this could be a matter of life or death'.[36] Even highly questionable 'addictions' are described in life-threatening terms. For example: 'Compulsive shopping can result in self-loathing, depression, financial ruin and marital breakups, yet often it is not considered a serious addiction . . . DON'T WAIT FOR DISASTER!'[37]

If the alcoholic, the overeater, the romantic, the Star Trekkie,[38] the market player[39] or the TV-watching couch potato claim they are not addicts, the Psychology Industry says they are in denial. The approach to dealing with denial is often coercive. The spouse is confronted with the choice of 'get help or I'm leaving', the employee with 'get help or you're fired', the accused with 'get help or go to jail'.

Unlike the early members of AA for whom their alcoholism was obvious, many of the new 'addicts' have to be persuaded to take the first step of admitting 'I am an addict.' Sometimes this is carried out in private sessions where problems are interpreted as 'symptomatic'. At other times it happens in support groups, as participants share their stories, accepting the newcomers as one of them. For instance, in AA, 'When newcomers claim that they cannot remember if they had any blackouts or not, other members use this claim as evidence of the event in question. As one member put it to a newcomer: "The reason you can't remember is because alcohol fogs your brain."'[40] Together, the psychologist and the group strive to establish the self-image of the person as an addict who, in turn, is a vulnerable, dependent and unfortunate victim.

Originally, AA was hostile towards medicine and psychology, but more recently a rapprochement has been arrived at whereby psychologists refer clients to the groups while the groups encourage individual treatment. They share a technology which some have equated to 'learning how to be an addict': acquiring the symptoms, accepting the identity and admitting the disease.

> *'We're all mad here. I'm mad. You're mad.'*
> *'How do you know I'm mad?' said Alice.*
> *'You must be,' said the Cat, 'or you wouldn't be here.'*
>
> Lewis Carroll, *Alice's Adventures in Wonderland*

For those who take on the new identity of a 'recovering addict', recovery is a never-ending process. For AA members, this means 'living one day at a time', 'improving their conscious contact with God', and spreading the 'spiritual awakening' to other alcoholics. For those in psychological treatment, this means living from one session to the next, developing a deeper psychological awareness and promoting their psychological awakening to other potential addicts. 'All of a sudden, people are pouring back into churches and synagogues,' writes one reporter.

> It appears that a great religious revival is sweeping the land – until you examine the situation a little more closely. Then you'll notice the biggest crowds today often arrive in midweek. And instead of filing into the pews, these people head for the basement, where they immediately sit down and begin talking about their deepest secrets, darkest fears and strangest cravings.[41]

Of this, Wendy Kaminer quips: 'never have so many known so much about people for whom they have cared so little.'[42]

Addiction treatment is a cash cow of the Psychology Industry, which has argued, in most cases successfully, that treatment of the 'disease' ought to be covered by health insurance. The state of Minnesota has declared alcoholism to be a treatable disease and adopted legislation against the firing of employees who are unable to perform their jobs because of drunkenness. They must be treated at the employer's (or insurer's) expense, even though most of the data show treatment to be ineffective. A survey of Fortune 500 companies indicated that 79 per cent recognized that substance abuse was a 'significant or very significant problem' in their organizations. However, when asked whether the treatment programmes did any good, 'the overwhelming majority saw few results from these programs. In the survey, 87 per cent reported little or no change in absenteeism since the programs began and 90 percent saw little or no change in productivity ratings.'[43]

Addiction treatment is a business whose failures lead to more business. Its technology, based on continued recovering, presumes relapses. Recidivism is used as an argument for further funding rather than as evidence of an ineffective treatment. The treatment business also actively recruits beyond the boundary of addicts, preaching the message that spouses are co-dependents and that children are highly susceptible to addiction. 'Children of alcoholics deserve and require treatment in and of themselves,' stated a founder of the National Association for Children of Alcholics.[44] It is also interesting to note that psychologist-assisted self-help groups, addressing addictions of all sorts, have become an adjunct treatment for many patients in therapy for nonaddictive problems. A recent study has shown that in a sample of women attending AA meetings, over half either didn't drink at all or weren't drinking heavily.[45] And Rutter, who specializes in the treatment of women with sexual-boundary issues (those he defines as sexually abused, by virtue of having had sex with a therapist, doctor, cleric, teacher etc.), recommends that his clients attend AA, Al-Anon or Adult Children of Alcoholic groups because 'the psychological dynamics of chemical dependency bear many similarities to those of sexual-boundary violations, and the two are often intertwined'.[46]

Noting how the Psychology Industry applies this technology to an endless host of new problems, John Leo whimsically writes that in 'this golden age of exoneration . . . Almost nobody can really be held accountable . . . Bonnie and Clyde came along too soon. Nowadays they could settle for a year at the Betty Ford Clinic as victims of compulsive bank-robbing addiction.'[47]

Trauma/Abuse

While addiction has been a significant aspect of the Psychology Industry for some time, trauma/abuse is a relatively new focus. Before the 1980s, trauma was generally associated with stress and treated as a medical problem. However, as Alice Miller and Jeffrey Masson championed the notion that psychological problems of adults were often due to bad or abusive parenting, and those involved in counselling Vietnam veterans promoted the concept of post-traumatic stress disorder (PTSD), a new enterprise was created: treatment technology for trauma/abuse.

Miller, a Swiss psychoanalyst, expressed the view that children are often exploited by parents and that society 'takes the side of the adult and blames the child for what has been done to him or her'. She argued that:

- The way we are treated as children is the way we treat ourselves the rest of our life.
- The child is always innocent.
- The child represses trauma and idealizes the abuser.
- This repression leads to neuroses, psychoses, psychosomatic disorders and delinquency.
- Therapy is successful only if the memories and feelings are uncovered.
- Fantasies serve to conceal truth but unconsciously convey childhood experience in symbolic ways.
- Past abuse can not be understood or excused as perpetrator's blindness or unfulfilled needs.
- Victims' reports can bring awareness and a sense of responsibility to society.[48]

Miller was vehemently critical of Freud and Freudians for what she considered to be a cover-up of the widespread social problem of child abuse.[49] Masson supported her claim when he printed letters purportedly showing that Freud altered his theory of incest to one of fantasy to protect his friend, Wilhelm Fleiss. He argued that this revision served to conceal the massive social problem of child abuse.[50]

The Miller/Masson theory was quickly accepted as a means to explain, via a single cause, a wide range of problems. But the application of their theory had an initial obstacle; many potential clients found it embarrassing and therefore hard to accept as an explanation of their own problems.

PTSD served to overcome that obstacle by casting the abuse theory within a broader, more palatable context. In discussing the 'advantages of using a PTSD diagnosis', Dolan writes:

> PTSD diagnosis is helpful for survivors of sexual abuse because the definition has a normalizing effect for clients . . . when symptoms of childhood sexual abuse are explained as initially reasonable, and in many cases, valuable efforts to survive extreme psychological stress, they become less stigmatizing in clients' eyes . . . Seeing themselves in the same group as victims of natural disasters, airplane and car accidents, and random criminal assaults can be helpful in overcoming a tendency to blame themselves rather than the perpetrator.[51]

This merger of the Miller/Masson theory with PTSD provided several advantages for the Psychology Industry:

- It's a simple, easily understood theory.
- The method is applicable to a wide range of problems and amenable to everyone, patient and psychologist alike.
- The treatment requires no previous training in psychology or psychiatry.
- It requires no knowledge of psychological assessment or psychi-

atric diagnosis, allowing traditional diagnostic categories to be ignored in favour of the all-inclusive label of PTSD.

FIGURE 2

T/A Technology

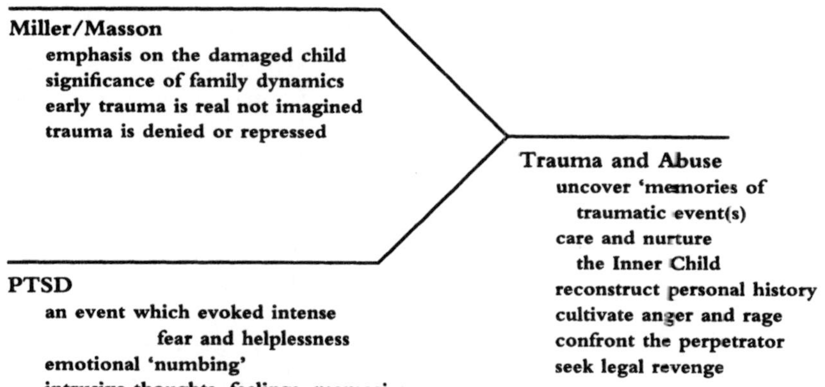

As McHugh notes, a patient's belief in trauma, abuse or incest 'makes psychotherapy seem easy. Therapists and patients can say: We have found the secret. The fact that patients and families steadily become more confused, incoherent and chaotic is accepted as an expression of the original incest.' But what really is happening, he says, is that 'conflicts are being generated by false memories. We have found something to make therapy easy.'[52]

'Once this diagnosis developed,' Blume writes, 'therapists independently began applying it to survivors of incest. Many have extended this application to other traumatized children: those who were physically, verbally, or sexually abused; those whose families were contaminated by alcoholism; those who witnessed the battering of a parent.'[53] And the list goes on, as concepts are stretched and treatments narrowed so that one size fits all. With a religious and moralistic zeal, psychologists have become aggressive, invasive and coercive in their style, some even claiming to have been 'anointed' by God.[54] Contrary to Dolan's view of 'normalizing', the application of PTSD has resulted in rampant pathologizing.

The success of this approach relies on the ability of psychologists to develop a victim identity in people with no idea that they have been abused. According to Blume, 'so few incest survivors in my experience have identified themselves as abused in the beginning of therapy that I have concluded that *perhaps half of all incest survivors do not remember* that the abuse occurred.'[55] Such syllogistic logic is evident in the bait-and-switch and misinformation tactics of many psychologists.

Williams describes how psychologists adopt the bait-and-switch tactics of retail sales practice in baiting clients by responding to their expectations of symptom reduction and emotional relief and, once they are hooked into treatment, telling them that their problems are deeper and more complex than they realize. They are then switched to the therapist's particular brand of treatment, which often takes longer and costs more.[56] To effect such switching, cognitive illusions are often relied on, such as:

> Victims of child abuse can't remember their early childhood.
> You can't remember your early childhood.
> Therefore, you must be a victim of child abuse.

This form of magical thinking gives the mistaken impression that unrelated variables are somehow connected, or that a symptom is proof of a cause. Frequently used checklists provide a similar function. For instance, Blume's 'Incest Survivors' Aftereffect Checklist', described as a 'standard diagnostic tool for clinicians and counsellors to identify incest survivors', begins with: 'Do you find many characteristics of yourself on this list? If so, you could be a survivor of incest,' and includes the following items:

4. Gastrointestinal problems; gynaecological disorders; headaches; arthritis or joint pain.

16. Trust issues: inability to trust; total trust; trusting indiscriminately.
23. Blocking out some period of early years (especially 1–12) or a specific person or place.[57]

Similarly, Whitfield provides a questionnaire including the following, which he claims 'reflects woundedness':

21. Have you tried counselling or psychotherapy, yet still feel that 'something' is wrong or missing?
24. Do you feel a lack of fulfilment in life, both personally and in your work?
30. Have you ever wondered if you might have been mistreated, abused or neglected as a child?[58]

And Jan Marie's list of thirty-one indicators of sexual abuse and incest includes such things as 'a dislike for tapioca pudding, mashed potatoes and runny eggs'.[59]

Whether through clinical suggestions or psychological quizzes and check lists, people are given the notion that their 'symptoms' are indicative of abuse or trauma. The next step is to solidify the victim identity by rehearsing, recovering and expanding memories of the event. So common is this process that Ganaway describes the trauma/abuse industry as 'memory mills with an almost assembly-line mentality'.[60]

'Memory work', as it is called by the Psychology Industry, is not only necessary to encourage clients to believe, it is essential to reinforce the victim state. Herman describes it as 'ambitious work. It requires some slackening of ordinary life demands, some 'tolerance for the state of being ill'.[61] 'The denial of an incest history must be broken through,' Blume declares, 'in order for healing to begin; one cannot recover from what one does not acknowledge and "breaking the secret" helps the survivor to acknowledge that she was unfairly harmed and is not a bad person . . . the more totally the previously buried traumas are uncovered and worked through, the deeper the recovery.'[62] Herman agrees: 'A narrative that does not include the traumatic imagery and bodily sensations is barren and incomplete.'[63] Within the Psychology Industry, there is a general consensus that memories, however arrived at, are requisite and the worse they are, the better.

Some psychologists, believing that these repressed memories are easily accessible through hypnosis, will simply ask the person what happened, who hurt them, how they were hurt. They accept the theory that traumatic memories are stored differently than other memories: sealed away in their original form, waiting for the safe moment to be accessed. Others practice a hypnotically induced 'age-regression', in which clients are led to believe that they are going back in time to their childhood. Frequently a mythical entity called by names, such as 'the Inner Child', 'the Child Within', 'the True Self', 'the Unconscious' or 'the Guide',[64] is called upon to assist in either 'finding' the memories or in uncovering the traumatic feelings imbedded in them. Based on pseudophilosophical theories of 'the innocent child', this entity is presumed to be the undamaged being who existed before the trauma and who continues to reside somewhere inside the person's unconscious, trapped by a cruel external world but desperately wanting to come out and be known, nurtured and protected.

> *'I can't believe that,'* said Alice.
> 'Can't you?' the Queen said in a pitying tone.
> 'Try again: draw a long breath, and shut your eyes.'
>
> Lewis Carroll, *Through the Looking-Glass*

When memories are sparse or when the psychologist, as in Gondolf's case, wants something more dramatic, other suggestive means are available. Maltz directs people who can't remember to 'spend some time *imagining that you were sexually abused*, without worry about accuracy or having your ideas make sense'. Others give clients the instruction to 'ground the experience or event in as much knowledge as you have and then let yourself *imagine what actually might have happened*'.[65] Cory Hammond, past president of the American Society of Clinical Hypnosis, presupposing abuse, will typically say to a person: 'You know, I know a secret about you.'[66]

On other occasions, psychologists rely on 'body memories' as the means to access lost information. Despite the lack of any research evidence to support the theory, Smith reports that in her survey of psychologists specializing in sexual abuse recovery, 59 per cent claimed that their clients experienced body memories and 95 per cent of the therapists said it was common for memories to surface via body memories.[67] Operating from this belief, many psychologists touch, massage or move their clients' bodies, watching for any reactions, memories or feelings that come to the client. Others practice 'somatic bridging', by asking clients to notice a feeling in the body and then let their minds follow that feeling back in time to another occasion when that feeling was stronger. One woman, who felt physically uncomfortable sitting in the chair, was instructed to 'follow that body feeling back in time'. Eventually she described a pain in her bottom which was interpreted as an early act of anal penetration.[68]

Not all trauma/abuse treatment consists of recovering memories; clients arrive with memories, both true and false. Often the therapeutic task involves reviewing and reinterpreting existing memories. Criticism from a boss is no longer merely uncomfortable; it is unrecognized abuse. The embarrassing comment of a father, the touch of a baby-sitter or the roughness of a physician's medical examination – all of these and many more can be transformed into trauma. Much of what the Psychology Industry does involves giving already existing memories new meaning, new character, new emotions and new importance.

Through the combination of biased interpretation, coercive suggestions and recovered memories, many can be persuaded that they are victims of trauma or abuse.[69] Herman claims that 'the traumatized person is often relieved simply to learn the true name of her condition. By ascertaining her diagnosis, she begins the process of mastery.'[70]

Adopting the victim identity is only the beginning; it takes practice to learn the intricacies of being a victim. As one of Hammond's patients said: 'I don't have that many memories. I'm new at this diagnosis.'[71] Another is quoted as telling a psychologist: 'Keep encouraging people to talk even if it's painful to watch them. It takes a long time to believe. *The more I talk about it, the more I have confidence that it happened,* the more I can integrate it. Constant reassurance is very important . . .'[72] Also considered important is the reconstruction of history, the identification of loss, the experience of grief and the expression of anger and rage.

For clients to become firmly set in their identity as victims, any prior sense of identity and trust must be shattered and replaced by a constructed life history of trauma, a story shadowed by fear and abuse. This 'new past' will be radically different from the one previously held, for 'if you maintained the fantasy that your childhood was "happy", then you have to grieve for the childhood you thought you had,' according to Bass and Davis.

> You must give up the idea that your parents had your best interests at heart . . . If you have any loving feelings toward your abuser, you must reconcile that love with the fact that he abused you . . . You may grieve over the fact that you don't have an extended family for your children, that you'll never receive an inheritance, that you don't have family roots.

This revised history becomes the foundation for the victim's identity and future; a dismal future as Nisbet predicts, for 'without roots, human beings are condemned to a form of isolation in time that easily becomes self-destructive.'[73] Since this reconstructed story is inevitably sad, the perceiving and telling of the story invariably 'plunges the victim into profound grief', which psychologists refuse to see for its destructive effect but rather as leading to 'the necessity of mourning . . . in the resolution of traumatic life events'. According to Herman, 'failure to complete *the normal process of grieving* perpetuates the traumatic reaction' for which the 'potential for pathological grief and severe, persistent depression is extremely high'. And Blume adds further emphasis: 'trauma theory addresses only part of the problem. Bereavement is necessary to address the other aspect of family trauma: the emotional loss suffered by the child . . . She grieves lost hopes, lost safety, lost innocence . . . Like the cognitive after-effects [of PTSD], grief is a normal and natural consequence of abuses such as incest.'[74]

In the Psychology Industry's technical guidebook, grieving leads directly to anger which must be developed and targeted at the perceived perpetrator, the family or anyone else deemed to have been complicit in the 'crime'. Clients are instructed 'to move . . . toward anger'[75] for 'anger is the backbone of healing'.[76] They are encouraged by psychologists to cultivate their rage:

> A little like priming the pump, you can do things that will get your anger started. Then, once you get the hang of it, it'll begin to flow on its own . . . Wanting revenge is a natural impulse, a sane response. Let yourself imagine it to your heart's content . . . Suing your abuser and turning him in to the authorities are just two of the avenues open . . . Visualize punching and kicking the abuser when you do aerobics . . . You can be creative with your anger . . . You can heal with anger.[77]

Anger and rage lead to 'empowerment', achieved through public recognition and retribution. According to Herman, 'the remedy for injustice also requires action'[78] – confrontation, litigation and social action. Since, by this time in the process, both the victim and the psychologist are convinced of the truth of the trauma, there is little hesitation about acting on the story as fact. Many are encouraged to confront their abuser as a means to gain this empowerment. They are told to 'Go in, say what you need to say, and get out.' In one example of such conducted confrontations, 'a woman went to her grandfather's funeral and told each person at the grave site what he had done to her. In Santa Cruz, California, volunteers from Women

Against Rape go with rape survivors to confront the rapist in his workplace.'[79]

Another suggested venue for confrontation is the courts.

> A lawsuit offers a survivor an opportunity to speak the truth about what happened, to break the silence. She is able to confront the person who abused her in a public forum, to seek *monetary compensation for therapy expenses*, lost income, and emotional distress, and to ensure that the abuser is confronted, in some way, with the effects of what he or she did.[80]

Although psychologists claim that knowledge is power, what they actually mean is that accusations render others powerless, entangled in a web of legal process and psychological absurdities. Herman endorses such legal action as a means of healing: 'by making a public complaint or accusation, the survivor defies the perpetrator's attempt to silence and isolate her, and she opens the possibility of finding new allies . . . the survivor may come to understand her own legal battle as a contribution to a larger struggle, in which her actions may benefit others as well as herself.'[81] While the overt and promoted benefits are incarcerated villains, vindicated victims and a revision of the legal system, the covert benefits are the further psychologizing of the law and society and an expanded market for psychologists to ply their wares. Although Bass and Davis admit that 'what lawsuits are best able to do is to get money',[82] they do not point out the major recipients of these funds are the lawyers and psychologists who build their career on victim-making.

While Freud has fallen into disrepute, the courts and the lawmakers have been persuaded to imbed some of his ideas into law, blurring legal concepts such as 'fact' and 'consent' with vague notions of 'recovered memories' and 'transference'. Just as 'memories' have been used to 'validate' claims of trauma and incest, so 'transference' has been used to establish abuse. One of the advocates of this trend is Peter Rutter, a Jungian analyst, consultant and expert witness on 'boundary issues', who views some of these psychologically determined laws as wonderful because they use the language of transference . . . a very real element that undermines the notion of free consent'.[83] According to Rutter, no longer can a woman function as a fully responsible and independent adult in any relationship with her male lawyer, doctor, therapist, cleric, teacher, mentor or other males, because 'the man holds in trust the intimate, wounded, vulnerable, or undeveloped parts of the woman'.[84] By this standard, women are considered to be naive, innocent and powerless, unable to assume the right and power to be responsible or self-determined. Although the stated goal is empowerment, its effect is that of disempowerment.

The Psychology Industry operates a powerful technology of victim-making. Sometimes the evoked emotionality of the users is mistaken for authenticity, and the emphatic statements of the psychologists for expertise; however, what their actions reflect is a simplistic process that ignores the individuality of people, the intricacies of thoughts and feelings, and the mysteries of the darker side of life. Ganaway's image of the assembly line seems fitting and raises other questions about the workers on the line.

Tailored (Taylored) Technicians

> *There is a serious dilemma occurring in our vocation and in our practice of helping people with their personal problems. The question is: are we training technicians or professionals?*
>
> Rollo May

The public's opinions and tastes are highly susceptible to commercial marketing whether in the form of direct advertising or indirectly through association with events and individuals. In the late 1990s, APA initiated an advertising campaign to shape public opinion about psychological services; they called it 'educating the public'. Although their specified goal was to stress the qualifications and expertise of licensed psychologists, setting them above others, the more likely effect will be to enhance the prestige of all those who sell psychological services, regardless of their training or licensing. The public is more susceptible to overall impressions than specific facts, to labels more than to descriptions of content, and is more likely to consider as the same all those who call themselves psychologists. Surveys have consistently shown that most people don't know the difference between psychiatrists, psychologists, psychotherapists and counsellors, presuming that they are all generally qualified, if for no other reason than that they say they are qualified. But are they?

An investigation of this question suggests that psychologists, regardless of what credentials they may or may not have, are *not* well trained, are often as badly off as their clients, apply their own values and ideas, however inappropriate, don't know or acknowledge their limitations, and get by either because they are just nice people or because they know how to play the role of an authority and expert.

Although the APA claims that there is 'value added when a mental health professional has at least a doctoral degree', this view expresses a bias which is supported neither by public opinion nor by empirical research. In response to a recent APA survey, only 29 per cent thought that a doctorate should be the minimum degree for treating depression, substance abuse or schizophrenia; 71 per cent did not share APA's view. And Dawes, in reviewing the literature on therapist effectiveness, concluded that 'there is no positive evidence supporting the efficacy of professional psychology'.[85] If this is so, then one would wonder why the APA argues differently, that psychology is 'a recognized and valued component of mainstream health care'.[86] The reason lies in society's move towards 'Taylored' mental health.

Taylorism was developed by Frederick Winslow Taylor, an early industrial psychologist. Early in the twentieth century, as the steel and automobile industries experienced labour strife related to factory mechanization and deplorable working conditions, he was hired to develop ways to control workers and boost their productivity. Taylor recognized that the specific knowledge and skill of workers, not possessed by management, gave employees power to control and limit production. So he proposed that management divide skilled work into its elementary component parts and redistribute it among workers, each of whom would perform limited tasks in ways rigidly defined by management (or indirectly defined by controls built into the machines they operate).[87] This change was perhaps most evident in the assembly-line technology developed by Henry Ford.

Taylorism offered a number of advantages to business: (1) it increased the dependence of workers and the power of management; (2) it lowered the cost of labour because unskilled people could be easily trained; (3) it allowed for easy replacement of 'troublemakers', and (4) it removed workers' freedom to influence production, making each worker, in Taylor's own words, 'a mere automaton, a wooden man'.[88] The relevance of Taylorism to the Psychology Industry is that it provides a model for the assembly-line approach to manufacturing and servicing victims which now characterizes much of American psychology.

Many of the effects of this Taylorism can now be seen within the Psychology Industry:

1. No longer does one have to have extensive academic training. If one can find a niche, one can be a recovered-memory therapist, addiction counsellor, CISD debriefer, victim services worker, assertiveness trainer, traumatologist; and the list goes on.
2. The economic effect of Taylorism was to lower the cost of labour. Now consumers can get therapy from these 'specialists' for much less than it would cost them to see a licensed psychologist. Seeing this as a means of lowering health-care costs, private, for-profit companies, referred to throughout the US as 'managed care organizations,' are hiring these 'specialists' and/or inviting previously employed licensed psychologists to put in bids for referrals.
3. Just as General Motors and Chrysler copied the assembly-line process of Ford, so have the various recovery therapies copied the twelve-step production process of AA. 'The American treatment of alcoholism follows a standard formula that appears

impervious to emerging research evidence (which shows no evidence of effectiveness), and has not changed significantly for at least two decades.'[89] The process is structured, leaving little room for variation or innovation. Thus, recovery therapies and many other psychological services have become Taylored rather than tailored to the needs of the individual.

Although many traditional psychologists are resisting the loss of their monopolistic power and protesting the reduction in their earnings, the door is now open, allowing those with limited skills, training and ability to be psychologists. Previously, a specialist was someone with additional training and advanced skills. However, 'Taylored psychology specialists' are different. They have a limited focus without the general training; they know less, not more. As Rollo May suspected, they are technicians disguised as professionals. Trained to see only through blinkered eyes, they are often unable to consider alternative diagnoses or treatments. Clients' problems are fitted to their limited skills, redefined according to their area of practice, and labelled with their particular approach in mind. Spiegel is outspoken about this when he says: 'the role of therapists in this whole phenomenon of multiple personality and victimization is more intriguing than the patients themselves. The therapists, with some exceptions, have become unconscious con artists. They are taking highly malleable, suggestible persons and molding them into acting out a thesis that they are putting upon them.'[90]

Consider the following testimony offered before a hearing into 'Violence and Abuse within the Family: The Neglected Issues,' sponsored by a Canadian senator:

In various legal contexts where abuse was the issue, evidence would be offered (in court) such as: the child was shy in the presence of the father, and that is indicative of child abuse. The child bed wet. The child's marks in school fell, or the marks rose; if they fell it was fear, if they rose it was because the school was an escape from the abuse. Either way, that was evidence of abuse.

> It becomes obvious that no matter what was observed, it was consistent with abuse. So you ask: 'What is inconsistent with abuse?,' and the answer always is: 'Well, nothing is inconsistent with abuse.' In fact, since most abused victims do not show any aftermath, the lack of symptoms itself is consistent with abuse. This is truly like falling into some kind of rabbit hole, like Alice in Wonderland. These 'child abuse experts' all share several things in common: first, they know nothing about science: they have no appreciation for concepts like 'control groups,' to make sure that suspected differences are objectively real and statistically significant: they have no idea at all that to learn something about a group, you have to study the 'not' group. Someone who only studies horses would tell you that the next creature with four legs is a horse because that's the only creature with four legs they have studied. And as a result, a lot of dogs will get saddled up in error.[91]

Some licensing boards are falling prey to this trend, issuing licences for limited scopes of practice to less educated groups. They expect these licensees to self-regulate, in other words, to restrict themselves from going beyond their skills; an amazingly foolish assumption by people who claim to understand human nature.

Who are these Taylored psychologists, these limited experts, these mental-health technicians? Williams, a psychologist, argues that some of them are the bait-and-switch operators who feed off of the public's assumptions and misperceptions about psychologists. Jay Schadler, a journalist, after watching hypnotists and recovered-memory specialists at work, thinks that 'some . . . may be as sick as their patients',[92] perhaps drawn into the business because of their own problems.

Alan Gold, a lawyer who has cross-examined psychologists in court for twenty years, thinks that some may lack the intelligence necessary to succeed in other fields. According to 'Gold's law', 'the "softer" the area of alleged expertise, the easier it is for dumbness to survive.' Citing Sykes's book *Dumbing Down Our Kids: Why American Children Feel Good About Themselves but Can't Read, Write or Add*, he continues: 'Dumbness does not last long in some industries, for example aircraft construction, where its mistakes crash and burn.' However, in the Psychology Industry, mistakes go unnoticed, failures are forgotten, and 'feeling good' is considered more important than thinking straight; all reasons Gold sees for 'why a growing population of high school educated "dummies" gravitate to therapy as a "profession"'.[93] He offers hundreds of case studies and court transcripts to support his theory.

One is left wondering, if some are slick and some are dumb, how are these Taylored psychologists able to function and, in doing so, persuade people of their importance and authority?

Although psychological technicians seem to be the way of the future for the Psychology Industry, the public continues to view psychologists as experts, setting them apart as authorities. The inducement towards imposture can be found in the professionally promoted notion that psychologists have superior knowledge, and in their own words, that they are 'experts in living'. Kottler, in his book *On Being a Therapist*, writes: 'Therapists have become the contemporary equivalent of the oracle perched on a mountaintop; clients are the pilgrims who journey in search of enlightenment. Mistrusting their own inner voices and lacking self-direction, clients look to their gurus for guidance and see them as embodiments of power to worship.'[94] And from his book *The Compleat Therapist*: 'It has become clear . . . that it hardly matters which theory is applied or which techniques are selected in making a therapy hour helpful . . . What does matter is who the therapist is as a human being – for what every successful healer has had since the beginning of time is charisma and power.'[95]

6
The Growth of the Psychology Industry

We must admit that the rapid growth of psychology in America has been due to conditions of the soil as well as the vitality of the germ.

J. M. Cattell, presidential address to the American Psychological Association, 1895

The growth of psychology as an industry in America is conveniently overlooked in most records of the history of psychology.[1] While it is true that, as a discipline, psychology has a rich philosophical and scholarly history, it is also true that a parallel history exists involving biased attention to whatever pays.

Throughout the history of civilization, the enquiring mind has been intrigued by its own workings and it was to this fascinating puzzle that psychology initially responded. However, this genuine inquisitiveness, along with objectivity and integrity, has succumbed to exaggerated claims, unsupported 'expert opinions', sweeping public statements, broad generalizations, fad treatments and trendy interest areas.

How did this happen? How did psychology reach this dubious point of becoming both an enormous industry within, and a product of, the society that it had promised to change?

To begin to understand this other history, one must consider the subtle but profound effects that nationalism, consumerism, feminism, genderism, professionalism and capitalism have had on what had begun as the science of psychology; how psychological 'facts' were created or distorted to support political or financial interests. Rather than the scientific approach of psychology being the correcting force, the Psychology Industry with its business plans, personal goals and social agendas has become the determining force shaping the profession. Although the academic discipline and the practice of psychology have had, until recently, quite separate and distinct histories, most people now use the terms synonymously. They view psychology as both a science that determines the 'facts' cited by psychologists, and a practice which involves the skillful and objective application of psychological knowledge. What virtually no one realizes is the extent to which the former has given way to the latter and, by aligning with other more powerful forces in society, fostered the growth of psychology into a major industry, thus sacrificing its soul (psyche) and its science (-ology).

Shaping and Being Shaped

Most people assume that the sciences are objective; concerned with fact and truth and not susceptible to the broader influences of society. But the sciences are as much *shaped* by the society in which they exist as they are *shapers* of that society. History is full of occasions when new discoveries were rejected because of the dogma of the times. As Schultz notes, 'even the greatest of minds (perhaps especially the greatest of minds) have often been constrained by what has been called the "Zeitgeist"';[2] that is, the general intellectual, moral and cultural climate of the era.

Similarly, most people, including most psychologists, assume that psychology serves society as a shaper. They fail to see that it has allowed itself to be shaped; to be influenced, restricted and directed by other forces in society in order to achieve its own prominence.

Regrettably, with what Rollo May calls 'the anti-historical tendency of psychology',[3] psychologists fail to acknowledge the relationship between their own aspirations for influence and affluence, and the effects of the political and social climate in which they work.

They tend to deny that their current theories and practices are the result of the interweaving of many historical, cultural and political factors which stretch well beyond the limited scope of psychology. With this arrogance ('what we "know" now is better than what they knew then') and denial ('what others think does not need to influence what we "know"'), psychologists ignore the past, placing the emphasis on what they call their 'new findings' and 'recent research'.

By disregarding history, they fail to see their transitory position in civilization. They do not wonder why it is that now, in the twentieth-century Western world, they have achieved recognition alongside medicine and law. They have not questioned their position in an industrial and capitalistic culture, nor their assumption that this society would provide the resources and the climate for a Psychology Industry to prosper. They have presumed that the power and policies of the United States would always favourably influence the international order, and that their place in the social fabric was secure. Like most in the Western world, they have grasped hold of an optimistic and opportunistic worldview that considers 'progress' to be onwards and upwards, bigger and better.

Despite their extravagant claims to understand people, they manifest an immense naivety about society which can only have profound implications for the nature of their theories of human behaviour. As Sarason writes: 'every psychologist has a picture of what man is or should be, of what society is or should be, and this picture infiltrates (indeed, is in part the basis of) his or her theories, along with the psychologist's way of thinking about theory and practice.'[4] Thus, what psychologists discover, promote or practise is also a product of their own wishes, goals and aspirations. They become agents of social influence and through their theories, expert opinions and work, they not only create a niche for themselves, they also advance their elitist, American image of the world which has shaped them.

If to be prominent is to be sensitive and responsive to the tides and whims of society, then to be successful is to merge one's personal goals with these larger social factors; to be a shaper who allows oneself to be simultaneously shaped.

Looking Back at the Past

Before the mid-1800s, psychology had been the province of philosophers and theologians, carried out through speculation and inference, intuition and generalization. However, by midcentury, the scientific method, which had shown modest gains in the understanding of physical nature, began to be applied to human nature. Even at this early stage, the foundation for a consumer-based psychology was being laid. Two interesting examples can be found in the area of intelligence testing, one of the first entrepreneurial activities of psychologists. The first provides an example of the misuse of science to support a psychologist's political beliefs; the second, perhaps more subtle in nature and profound in its eventual effect, demonstrates the susceptibility of a psychologist to the dominant values inherent in his society.

Sir Francis Galton, well known in the history of psychology and a cousin of Charles Darwin, sought to apply the theory of evolution to that of intellectual capacity. In 1869 he published *Hereditary Genius*, which held that eminent men have eminent sons; that is, that intellectual greatness is inherited.[5] To 'prove' his assumptions, Galton studied the ancestries of famous scientists, jurists, physicians and the like, individuals of genius and all members of the aristocracy. His ultimate goal was to encourage the production of the more eminent or mentally fit and to discourage the birthrate of those deemed unfit. Galton had not only wanted to understand the inherited quality of greatness; he also wanted to use psychology to protect and maintain the power of his social class which was under threat of change. Britain's position as a world power was being challenged. The dominant aristocratic class feared being replaced by the rising class of unsophisticated but wealthy financiers and industrial barons. In defence of political inequity, he declared: 'The average citizen is too base for the everyday work of modern civilization' and all citizens are therefore not 'equally capable of voting'. This inequality carried with it social consequences which Galton made explicit: lower-class citizens should be treated with kindness only 'so long as they maintained celibacy', but if they 'continued to procreate children, inferior in moral, intellectual and physical qualities, it is easy to believe that the time may come when such persons would be considered as enemies to the State and to have forfeited all claims to kindness'.[6] Under the guise of protecting society, he established the Eugenics Laboratory at University College, London, and founded an organization to promote ideas of racial improvement and the supremacy of the gifted.

From the vantage point of the late 1990s, with the intervening history of the Holocaust, Stalinism and the repeated reports of cultural and racial 'cleansing', one would wonder how this attitude could have been held by one as prominent and respected as Galton. However, his work bore the imprint of his social class and in the end it 'proved' what he and they wanted to believe: that intelligence was genetically inherited and that psychological technology must be employed to protect and improve it. And this view was not restricted to England. As Hernstein and Murray noted, regarding the United States:

> The first wave of public controversy occurred during the first decades of the century, when a few testing enthusiasts proposed using the results of mental tests to support outrageous racial policies. Sterilization laws were passed in sixteen American states between 1907 and 1917, with the elimination of mental retardation being one of the prime targets of the public policy. 'Three generations of imbeciles are enough,' Justice Oliver Wendell Holmes declared in an opinion upholding the constitutionality of such a law. It was a statement made possible, perhaps encouraged, by the new enthusiasm for psychological testing.'[7]

In the same time period, in France, Alfred Binet was studying the intellectual development of children. Unlike Galton, who viewed formal schooling as a waste of money because intelligence was inherited, Binet believed that education appropriate to ability could prepare children for the emerging industrial society. To help reform the public school system, he developed a scale to measure intelligence, a concept which he interpreted as the ability to solve certain types of logical problems. It was this definition of intelligence, influenced by the attitudes and needs of an industrialized society, that lead Sarason to comment about Binet: 'his world view prevented him from recognizing that his concept of intelligence was an invention and, like all inventions, as revealing of the inventor's society as of the inventor.'[8]

This scale may have been the first successful product of the Psychology Industry as it merged the needs of an industrializing society with the aspirations of the psychologist; and it marked the beginning of the phenomenal growth of mental testing. Binet's scale and the whole concept of mental testing was quickly seized upon and applied with eagerness particularly by American psychologists, who saw it as a way to establish the importance of psychology. American society wanted a practical, down-to-earth form of psychology, and mental testing provided the first of many ways that psychology could be used in a bold and direct American way.[9] As well as assisting the government in making political and racial decisions, such as the barring of 'defective aliens', it provided industry with a means to select and train workers. Like Binet, these early entrepreneurial psychologists failed to consider, or refused to acknowledge, how their definition of intelligence really expressed the values of their affluent social class; one being that intelligent people make better citizens and better workers.

These examples are not intended to suggest the existence of any malevolence or sinister conspiracy. Rather, they serve to demonstrate that, from the beginning, psychology has furthered its own interests by yielding objectivity and responding to the demands and beliefs of its own social world, often failing to go far enough in its thinking and questioning. 'The inability of these psychologists to ask and pursue questions insured that their theories and research would play into and reinforce the prejudiced attitudes of the dominant groups in society, groups to which these psychologists belonged'[10] – a characteristic evident now in the Psychology Industry.

Following Medicine's Example

Psychology was neither alone nor the first to exploit social opportunities. Medicine had chosen the same route and led the way both in professionalization, which restricted the competition and established control over the market, and in developing a mutually beneficial working relationship with business and industry. Medicine became the model that the Psychology Industry followed in building itself as a competitive business.

Before the mid-1800s, the state of medicine in North America, as practised by pharmacists, homeopaths, osteopaths, herbalists, local shamans and some regular doctors with what then passed for medical training, was so abysmal that patients with cholera were given an even chance of being done in by the disease or by the doctor.[11] However, in the latter half of the century, American medicine began to adopt a scientific approach as it studied the body, created esoteric diagnoses and developed technical treatments.

Scientific medicine served the needs of the financiers and industrialists; it was politically and economically useful to the affluent capitalist class. To ensure its viability, a number of wealthy industrialists, led by Andrew Carnegie and John D. Rockefeller, developed a form of philanthropy that built and endowed medical schools which agreed to technically train and properly socialize their students. In turn, this benefited the doctors who, rewarded with professional prestige and influence, gained control over their competition. Through the joint efforts of the American Medical Association and industry, laws came to be enacted that restricted medical licensing to scientifically trained practitioners and penalties were established for even fraternizing with the unlicensed.

This self-serving relationship, which allowed business interests to determine how doctors should think, and whom and what they should treat, shaped not only the practice of medicine but eventually also the practice of psychology, for it was from within medicine that the current practice of the Psychology Industry emerged.

The medical literature of the 1800s abounded with descriptions of neurasthenia, hysteria and hypochondriasis, as well as lunacy and insanity. The psychological symptoms they presented could be detected in people's mood and behaviours. These conditions were spoken of as 'shattered nerves',[12] a term reflecting the belief that they were due to physical problems in the nervous system. The most severe instances were treated by 'mad doctors' who worked behind high walls in insane asylums. However, as cases were identified among members of the wealthier upper class who desired to avoid the embarrassment of incarcerating a family member, a new designation of medical specialist developed, the 'alienist' (from the phrase 'alienation of the mind'). These doctors focused on a broader range of problems which fell under the title of 'mental pathology' or 'medical psychology'.

It was from this that Sigmund Freud, a neurologist by training, developed the field of psychoanalysis. Among Freud's notable contributions was his description of the unconscious, a concept of which many, including the hypnotists, were already aware,[13] and his explanation of family dynamics, including the contentious theory of infantile sexuality which still plays a role in the internal disputes of the Psychology Industry. Freud saw psychoanalysis as a means of understanding the dark side of human nature and he believed that increased understanding by the individual could lead to greater acceptance of one's self and to a reduction in anxiety, considered to be the result of unconsciously trying to hide these less flattering, darker aspects.

Although the medical establishment in Europe was sceptical, psychoanalysis was quickly and eagerly picked up and Americanized by the fledgling psychiatric profession in the United States who saw it as a means to mould or adapt the individual to the changing world. G. Stanley Hall, the host for his 1909 visit to America, told Freud that he had come at a good 'psychological moment',[14] a time when, 'with mobility of place, profession and status, and a new instability of values, old ways of looking at the world no longer applied. The individual is thrown back on himself and is more receptive to theories such as psychoanalysis which search for meaning in his dreams, wishes, fears, and confusion.'[15] By acquiring psychoanalysis, watering it down and sweetening it to their taste, American psychiatrists brought 'Freudianism in line with American beliefs about the virtue and necessity of an optimistic approach . . . and promised that self-improvement was possible without calling society into question'.[16] Americanized psychoanalysis defined psychological problems as being specific to the individual, reducing any broader social context such as alienation, poverty or industrialization. Now, eighty years later, American psychology has a similar character, emphasizing individual issues and ignoring the larger social context.

Transformed into a formal American institution, psychoanalysis served the mutual interests of the individual, society and medicine. For the person experiencing the instability of an external world in which the old way did not apply, it offered a means to search for personal meaning in dreams, fantasies, fears and anxiety. For the industrialized society, it taught people that problems and solutions were to be found inside one's self and not in the external world. And for psychiatrists, who imported the theory and protected its esoteric language (e.g. catharsis, id, abreaction), it provided both the theory and procedures that made them distinct from, but acceptable to, their medical colleagues. The decision of the American Psychoanalytic Association, in 1927, to limit the practice of psychoanalysis to medical doctors served to further its medicalization, its professionalization and the elite status of its members as psychological specialists. By maintaining their medical identity, analysts adopted a pseudo-scientific stance and generally ignored the metaphorical, poetic and 'magical' aspects inherent in its nature when Freud and Jung first conceived it.

American psychoanalysis became preoccupied with a picture of the psyche which emphasized the ego and its healthy ability to control and master conflicts and urges. Basically it supported and promoted the optimistic American dream of health, wealth and happiness. The French analyst Jacques Lacan described the American psychoanalytic movement as offering 'to the Americans to guide them towards happiness, without upsetting the autonomies, egotistical or otherwise, that pave with their non-conflictual spheres, the American Way of getting there'.[17] Psychoanalysis had secured a place for itself in American culture, appearing to meet the demands for therapeutic and medical precision, to give meaning and hope for change, and to do it without challenging or upsetting the social order.

Just as psychoanalysis sought to maintain its connections with scientific medicine, psychology claimed the nature and measurement of behaviour as its domain of scientific expertise. This approach provided a subject amenable to laboratory study and of interest to business and industry. The gain for medicine and psychology was not only professional status, but social prestige, a monopoly on practice and increased influence. What aspects of these relationships were conscious and what were unconscious is not the issue here. What is, is that both groups had aligned with dominant forces (i.e. the shapers) existing in their world and in so doing had opened themselves to the influence of these powers (to be 'shaped'). As Brown writes: 'the obvious advantages to the profession(s) notwithstanding, scientific medicine (and one can add psychology) contained within it the seeds of ultimate destruction for the profession.'[18]

The Fertile Soil

Why was the United States so ready to accept psychology?

In part, America was ripe for all sciences, whether they were natural, like physics and biology, or social, like psychology and political science. 'Americans possessed a very high regard for science,' Kurt Koffka observed, '"accurate and earthbound" science, which produced in them an aversion, sometimes bordering on contempt, for metaphysics that tries to escape from the welter of mere facts into a loftier realm of ideas and ideals.'[19]

In academia, psychology had won its independence from philosophy and was becoming identified as the source of new behavioural techniques which would lead society 'on its onward and upward course to human betterment'.[20]

Meanwhile the advent of monopolistic capitalism, in which larger industries swallowed up the smaller, was resulting in fewer but larger groups of workers who now had the ability and the strength to object to their conditions of work, to disrupt production and to cause industrial unrest. It was to psychology that industry appealed for solutions, encouraging those like Taylor to develop methods to control and manipulate the labour force.

Notable is the work of Elton (George) Mayo, an Australian psychologist brought to the United States by the Rockefeller Foundation. His well-known research at the Hawthorne Plant of the Western Electric Company, although severely flawed and later judged to be invalid, had a profound and lasting effect on industry and on the whole of applied psychology.[21] His conclusion was that workers have an 'eager desire for cooperative activity' and function better in groups, rather than as isolated individuals. He believed that the 'Hawthorne effect', as it came to be known, provided conclusive evidence that 'friendly supervision' led to greater productivity and less unrest without the employer having to concede any costly improvements in wages or working conditions. As a result, Mayo claimed to have discovered a new method of human control: 'the power of human relations'.[22]

Despite the shoddy research,[23,24] Mayo's work had two profound effects which would later spread from industry to the psychotherapeutic community: the invention of the 'non-directive' interviewing technique and the genesis of the 'human-relations movement'. Mayo taught interviewers to listen attentively without interrupting, focusing on the workers' personal situations rather than on their work grievances. This non-directive style served as a powerful emotional release of resentment. It also implied that the company had concern for the workers' feelings, and fostered a rapport or cooperative relationship between the workers and the company. Although termed 'non-directive,' it was blatantly controlling since it defined workers' problems as originating within themselves rather than from any common workplace issues. An example of this co-opting power comes when a worker makes the general statement that the piece rates on his job are too low. In the interview, he reveals that his wife is in hospital and that he is worried about the doctor bills he has incurred. The interviewer is able to refocus the complaint so that it consists of the fact that his present earnings, due to his wife's illness, are insufficient to meet his current financial obligations.[25] Such an inner-directing approach was enthusiastically adopted by industry, and the Rockefeller and Ford foundations generously funded Carl Rogers to refine this human-relations technique, which would later, through similar use with university students, emerge as Rogerian psychotherapy.

In spite of the lack of any valid or reliable scientific basis, the philosophy of Mayo and his associates became the foundation of the human-relations approach that would dominate industry through the 1940s and 1950s. In a peculiarly American way, it held the optimistic view that individuals were naturally energetic, industrious and achievement-oriented. Those workers who failed to produce or who disrupted the 'friendly relationship' were judged to have a personal problem. It emphasized structured counselling techniques to develop positive mental attitudes, an approach that would become the basis for the humanistic psychotherapy movement of the 1960s and 1970s. And it created a new occupational category: interviewer/counsellor, which would, in time, lead to the growth of nonprofessional counsellors and psychotherapists.

Behaviourism

With the shift away from the exploration of consciousness to the focus on behaviour and performance, it was natural to study the behaviour that was being observed and measured.

Ivan Pavlov, the Russian physiologist, had demonstrated that since dogs would quite naturally begin to salivate when shown food, if a bell was rung when the food was given, the sound of the bell could cause the dogs to produce saliva even when there was no food.[26] In Pavlov's thinking, this 'conditioned reflex' was the result of a physiological connection (an 'arc') inside the brain. Unconcerned with such physiological explanations, John B. Watson, often called the father of behaviourism,[27] insisted that psychology address only 'the prediction and control of observable behaviour', abandoning any and all interests in mental and body states, instincts, introspection or any other 'ghosts in the machine' as he called them. In contrast to the earlier focus of psychology on abilities and traits, Watson's behaviourism saw all behaviours, which he called 'responses', as a result of outside 'stimuli', susceptible to being developed, managed and controlled by external forces.[28] Watson urged psychologists to focus on 'the problems of living . . . and to deal with matters of practical consequence, such as the psychology of advertising, and of testing . . .'[29]

When Watson experienced a sudden fall from grace in the academic community because of a sensationalized divorce, he quickly found his place in a receptive advertising industry, where he remained, with success, until his retirement. 'In this pursuit he had the company of A. A. Brill, who used his psychological expertise to develop advertising that encouraged women to smoke. Psychology was used by business to ensure that consumption kept pace with production.'[30] Behaviourism also developed a wider political effect as it became a means to influence and control various groups in society. For example, Watson applied his popular ideas to such social topics as child-rearing, writing that children could be conditioned for either genius and success, or 'doltishness' and failure. In contrast to the permissive, developmental approach of the psychoanalysts, he believed that it was the parents' responsibility to provide the appropriate conditions to ensure the proper upbringing and, with this, anything was possible.[31]

Psychology and the Military

In the years leading up to the First World War, the procedures of psychological measurement, begun in the perception labs of Weber, Wundt and Helmholz in Germany, and in the work of Galton and Binet, flourished. Psychologists such as Cattell began to measure all sorts of abilities and functions in order to determine human capacity and to identify individuals with disabilities. So apparently successful was the venture that both government and industry expressed interest and encouragement for the development of psychological tests for military and vocational selection. Whether it was to produce good soldiers or good workers, the intention was the same: to develop the means through which the 'human machine' could be made to function most efficiently. Funding from such sources provided psychologists with a further opportunity to promote their profession. Such intentions are evident in the vote of the Council of the APA in 1917:

> To appoint committees from the membership of the American Psychological Association to render to the government of the United States all possible assistance with psychological problems arising from the present military emergency . . . American psychologists can substantially serve the government under the medical corps of the Army and Navy by examining recruits with respect especially to intellectual deficiency, psychopathic tendencies, nervous instability and inadequate self-control . . .[32]

Psychologists, while appearing to respond to a call for patriotism, were moving to assert themselves as essential to their society. By assuming the role of identifying and weeding out mental incompetents and disruptive individuals, psychologists were allying themselves with the stronger forces of government. The commentator Walter Lippman expressed his concern at the time when he wrote of the power-hungry intelligence testers who yearned to 'occupy a position of power which no intellectual has held since the collapse of theocracy',[33] but no one heeded the warning.

For the first time, the government became actively involved in applying psychology on a mass scale to the armed forces.[34] Such an opportunity provided an 'ideal laboratory' in which to study large numbers of people in a controlled environment and to develop techniques which would later prove useful to, and be used extensively by, industry. Interestingly, it was from this experience, and with these tools, that the Psychological Corporation was started in 1921 by Cattell, funded by $10 shares bought by APA members, for the purpose of promoting the application of psychology. It remains one of the major international suppliers of psychological tests for use in industry, education and clinical treatment.

The Second World War posed similar problems for the United States and its allies, who needed both to produce and maintain strong soldiers and strong workers, and to influence public opinion. Again psychology responded, not only with the traditional huge screening programmes to select personnel, but also with services which relied on its experience in advertising: attitude formation, propaganda techniques and analysis, and counter-intelligence. In addition, it began to do something with which it was totally unfamiliar and inexperienced: to treat psychological casualties. As members of the military, psychologists studied the behaviour of soldiers under varying degrees of stress and their findings led to treatment innovations including group therapy, brief therapy, hypnosis and stress management techniques, all aimed at improving the efficiency of normal people under stress and getting soldiers back into conflict.

A significant shift was taking place. Psychologists were beginning to treat 'normal people with problems'. The market for their services expanded significantly as they defined a much larger group as being in need of treatment. Through the efforts of William C. Menninger, a prominent industrial psychiatrist[35] and the director of the US Army psychiatric programme, the first version of the *Diagnostic and Statistical Manual (DSM)* was created which gave far more recognition and emphasis to the 'neuroses' and behavioural problems which plagued both business and the military. By classifying problems in this way, the *DSM* further established them as being the appropriate concern and territory for the Psychology Industry.[36] It was becoming clear that psychologists viewed therapy as a legitimate aspect of their professional role, second only to assessment.[37]

By the end of the war in 1945, psychology had become well established in identifying and treating those individuals who either failed to conform or to be productive according to the capitalistic American model. Psychologists were convinced that they had much to contribute in building the postwar world, through policy and research and through training others in applied psychology. Psychology was clearly accepting and promoting its double identity as a science and as a technological means to better the world which saw itself emerging into a victorious and optimistic future.

The Promise of Psychology

The postwar growth of psychology was comparable only to the optimistic and excited reception it received from all aspects of society. The scientism of psychology made grand promises: solutions to societal and international problems, understanding and change of individual and social behaviour, and the creation of a safer and better world by eliminating the destructive forces that had brought about the war so that war would have no place again. 'If the weltanschauung of psychology changed in the two decades after World War II, it was in the strengthening of the axiom that the social world is knowable, predictable, and controllable and in the related axiom that breakthroughs in understanding the individual human mind would be basic building blocks for a better society.'[38] Applied programmes of psychology were started in universities, clinical departments were created in hospitals, research funds were poured into the social sciences and government agencies were established to study mental health.[39] 'The purists were a minority. Here and there they were able to keep their enclaves pure, but overall the integration between the hard- and the soft-headed came about . . . by the pressure of external society and fatefully, federal money. Psychology as a science and practice were married.'[40] The disparate parts of psychology were merging to form the Psychology Industry.

Probably the most prominent aspect of postwar psychology and the most relevant to the developing Psychology Industry was the revision of behavioural psychology by B. F. Skinner.[41] His interest was to describe and predict behaviour, not to explain it with what he called 'spurious physiologizing'. He had no interest in exploring the attitudes and beliefs, the dreams and fears inside the person. The individual came to be considered as an 'empty-organism' or a 'black box', of interest only for what external behavioural responses it emitted.[42] Skinner believed that behaviour was more directly related to the outcome or the effect it produced; the 'reinforcement', as he termed it. And like Thorndike half a century earlier, he believed that those behaviours which led to satisfaction (i.e. positive reinforcement) would increase in probability.

Known as 'operant conditioning', Skinner's concepts became widely popular, appearing in education (teacher-training methods), psychiatric treatment (token economies), therapy (desensitization and behaviour modification) and business (reinforcement scheduling). Psychoanalytic treatment had been popular immediately after the war but was superseded by the quicker and surer change promised by the behaviourists regardless of personality characteristics or family upbringing.

The applied products of behavioural psychology became a technological foundation for industry. The model assumed that people can and should be made to adapt to a relatively unalterable world. Whether as children, patients or employees, they were rewarded or reinforced for behaviours that were considered appropriate by the teacher, psychologist or employer. Behaviour modification seemed to be a godsend. It was cheaper, faster and more reliable in moulding new behaviour. It was easy to teach, so behaviour therapists could be produced quickly from the pool of untrained personnel. It required no trust, rapport or friendliness. And it made obedience or conformity its goal, not the 'insight' of psychoanalysis or the 'happiness' of human relations. It was ideal for the school, the factory, the home; for the whole of a controlling society. Its popularity grew, and with it grew the Psychology Industry.[43]

Psychology was in its heyday. In 1955, Fillmore Sanford, the executive secretary of the APA, predicted: 'If the present rate of growth continues, we will have, by simple arithmetic, 60 million members 100 years from now; and in 200 years, if we continue to grow, membership in the association will coincide exactly with membership in the human race.' Considering the current cultural susceptibility to psychological ideas, the prediction may not have been as absurd as it sounds.

However, it was from this time that psychology as a science began a rapid decline while schools of clinical and applied psychology virtually exploded in number. Licensing laws were introduced and passed in state after state, ostensibly to protect the public from unqualified practitioners but in actuality creating publicly sanctioned, monopolistic professions. Psychology as a science was being replaced by psychology as an industry. Psychologists were discovering that they could earn far more in business than they could in the university. The results of research now became the fodder for therapeutic theories and health-promotion programmes.

This was already evident in the behaviourism movement. The empirical approach of the laboratory flowed into the consulting room where psychologists offered 'scientific' treatment approaches based on the principles of classical (Pavlovian) and operant (Skinnerian) conditioning with such labels as 'behaviour modification', 'systematic desensitization' and 'behaviour therapy'.[44] Rapid and effective treatment was promised for the 'anxiety neuroses' of the day, which had replaced the 'repressive disorders' prominent in Victorian society. Psychological treatment was now available without need for medical diagnoses ('the symptom is the disease') or stigma. New and wannabe psychologists were able to learn and dispense simple and easily understandable concepts without the requirement of extensive professional training. With this new category of behaviour therapist, a form of psychological Taylorism was beginning which would grow in the decades to come. By the middle of the 1960s, the behavioural orientation had gained wide acceptance with 'scientifically proven' results and was being promoted to mental-health workers, educators and physicians. It was even suggested that the blessings of behavioural technology 'may be the elimination of mental illness, crime and even war'.[45]

However, some critics expressed concern that psychology and its technologies were becoming the sources of social control, discouraging or diverting people from 'seeking solutions that work, solutions that might be disturbing to the social, economic and political status quo'.[46]

The Boom and the Desperation

The latter part of the 1960s marked a radical change in psychology and in the nature of the Psychology Industry, in part owing to economic factors and in part to the social and political climate. It was becoming clear that the long-term viability of the industry rested on third-party recognition of psychologists as reimbursable providers of 'medical' services. Through the organized lobbying activities of the professional associations, the public gained greater access to psychological services.[47] Socially, the physical sciences and technology had created a more comfortable, if not happier, world to live in and had contributed a plethora of 'time-saving' and 'leisure-enjoying' devices. American society enjoyed wealth in leisure and money beyond anything previously experienced. However, it failed to achieve the emotional and social benefits of peace, security and safety. Internationally, the threat of a nuclear holocaust hovered as the war in Vietnam demonstrated technological disregard for human life (both friend and foe). Domestically, people sensed that they had lost control of corporations and that these giants now controlled American society.

From this discontent, a significant and vocal minority, the hippies, emerged with their counterculture. They challenged the values and benefits of the technological society. As the historian Theodore Roszak stated then:

> from my point of view, the counter culture, far more than merely 'meriting' attention, desperately requires it, since I am at a loss to know where, besides among these dissenting young people and their heirs of the next few generations, the radical discontent and innovation can be found which might transform this disoriented civilization of ours into something a human being can identify as home.[48]

The thrust of technology 'to know' was challenged by the call of the hippies 'to live'. For them, 'the primary purpose of human existence [was] not to devise ways of piling up ever greater heaps of knowledge, but to discover ways to live from day to day that integrated the whole of our nature by way of yielding nobility of conduct, honest fellowship, and joy.'[49]

A psychologist who provided impetus to the counterculture and encouraged the emergence of a pop philosophy of psychotherapy was Fritz Perls. Introducing gestalt therapy to the human-potential enthusiasts of the late 1960s, he became an icon of the 'personal growth' movement, which was by then the public outgrowth of industry's human-potential movement. It was Perls who coined the hippie term 'mind-fucking' to describe what he perceived as the controlling nature of psychoanalysis and other verbal therapies. Blatantly romantic, he and his associates promoted the belief that within everyone is the potential for emotional stability and happiness, achievable through gestalt therapy. Optimism was for sale.

The Psychology Industry took this as an opportunity for innovation and expansion. Three main changes occurred in the psychology business at this time: (1) the technical definitions of psychology and psychotherapy were expanded to include a variety of unusual and quasi-therapeutic techniques; (2) technology was broadened so that what constituted 'good' psychology became an open-ended question; and (3) training options proliferated so that who was a 'qualified' psychologist became less clear and the therapeutic marketplace became more competitive than ever before.[50] Academic psychology and the profession of psychiatry lost their hold on the Psychology Industry as the market became flooded with techniques ranging from transactional analysis, hypnosis, existential analysis, Rolfing and primal therapy to re-evaluation therapy, est, Reichian sensitivity, bioenergetics and journeys into consciousness.

In a move to detach and distinguish themselves from their conservative and conforming scientific predecessors, psychologists now promoted the goal of 'growth' rather than 'cure'. Grasping the vast opportunities, they began to echo the words of Erving and Miriam

Polster: 'Therapy is too good to be limited to the sick.' It was readily accepted, bought and paid for by 'an educated public eager for some easy form of psychological salvation in which you didn't have to be sick in order to get well.'[51] Gone (temporarily) was the medical view of therapy and in its place, a populist version arose in which 'being in therapy' was something about which to be proud and public. Traditional training in psychology was no longer a prerequisite for the successful development of a psychotherapy practice. In fact, some began to argue that formal training might actually impair an individual's natural abilities for helping and that it was easier and better to train therapists without worrying about their knowledge of medicine, psychology, social work or counselling.[52] As Perry London commented, all one really needed to 'establish one's own [psychology] business, and bona fides, [was] the right blend of nerve and entrepreneurial skill'.[53] Relevant personal experience ('you have to have been there yourself to help others') also became an important quality of the 'good' psychologist; a belief that would spawn the growth of the self-help movement in the 1980s and become an apparent requirement of the recovery therapists of the 1990s.

While group treatment had existed for as long as individual psychotherapy, its economic benefits (i.e. one psychologist and more patients, paying lower fees per person) became obvious with the growth in demand for psychological services. Within the hippie humanitarian concept of fellowship, the psychologist became the first among equals and enjoyed a larger income while serving more people. It was not a big step from this happy juncture of profit and productivity to the marathon or 'group intensive' sessions which functioned as pressure cookers to force regression, which appeared as irrational expressions of emotions.[54] And from this, the approach expanded to the weekend experience and the therapeutic workshops and seminars of the 1980s and 1990s in which a short piece of work could result in an even larger net profit.

This 'me first' form of psychotherapy was not restricted to the left-wing and hippie groups; establishment versions were developed and provided by psychologists employed by industry. Reminiscent of Mayo's human-relations movement, sensitivity or T-groups, as they were known, promoted 'closeness, trust, authenticity and confrontation', with the expressed aim that 'healthier executives' made better managers who could better achieve the corporate goals. All aspects of business, including education, health, the private sector and government, bought into this new form of human relations. Between 1968 and 1970, the US Department of Labor alone spent $1.44 million to teach sensitivity to its supervisors.

It would be incorrect to assume that all of the psychology vendors at this time were frauds or charlatans or that all of the customers were merely gullible. What is accurate is that both were willing parties, invested in their own self-interests and each seeing the other as a means to achieve these goals. The customers pursued their mythical American goals of 'love', 'self-actualization', 'awareness' and 'higher consciousness', while the Psychology Industry built its therapeutic metropoles and merchandised 'growth services'.

At a Boulder, Colorado, conference on graduate education in clinical psychology, Victor Raimy declared: 'Psychotherapy is an undefined technique applied to unspecified cases with unpredictable results. For this technique, rigorous training is required.'[55] By the end of the 1970s, Herink reported that the number of name-brand psychotherapies exceeded 250.[56]

These subjective, sometimes poorly articulated and generally non-establishment approaches might have continued for generations were it not for changes occurring within psychology and within the larger social context. The general popularity of psychology had grown exponentially, resulting in aggressive competition for market share. No longer was there any shortage of psychologists. However, the boom in health care and social welfare spending of the affluent 1960s and early 1970s was coming to an end as costs were exceeding all budgets.

The US Health Maintenance Organizations (HMOs) Act of 1973 specifically required funds for mental-health services, including out-patient and substance-abuse treatment. Intended to control spiralling health costs, HMOs were able to slow down the inflationary increases of medicine and surgery. However, mental-health costs went out of control, with inpatient costs accelerating at three times the inflation rate of medical and surgical costs.[57] The response of HMOs was to impose accountability, including requirements on psychologists to demonstrate cost-effectiveness.

The Psychology Industry had always concluded that psychotherapy was effective despite the lack of research evidence to support this assumption. Outcome evaluations and cost–benefit studies suggested, at best, that psychotherapy was somewhat effective with some of the clients some of the time. Parloff, in reviewing nearly 500 rigorously controlled studies, concluded that 'the research evidence . . . has not met the needs of the policy makers and does not greatly enhance the credibility of the field of psychotherapy.'[58] While there may have been scientific literature to support the efficacy of psychotherapy in very well-controlled laboratory contexts, there was no evidence that the effects were the same in the real world.

This discouraging situation led Seligman, in 1995, to introduce his 'gold standard' measure of consumer satisfaction. In his APA presidential column in December 1998, he admits that 'specific [psychotherapy] effects are hard to find', and he suggests that the effects of therapy are due to what he calls 'tactics' and 'deeper strategies'. As tactics, he names 'attention, authority figure, rapport, alliance, tricks of the trade (e.g., "Let's pause here," rather than "Let's stop here"), paying for services, . . .' which sound like the characteristics one might attribute to successful faith healers and salesmen. As 'strategies' he includes those which help to build courage, interpersonal skills, rationality, optimism, capacity for pleasure and honesty.[59] While these may be desirable human strengths, encouraging them hardly seems to be an identifiable skill to which any profession might legitimately lay claim.

Understandably, insurers and other funding sources have not been favourably impressed with all these excuses to deal with the lack of demonstrable effectiveness. In the 1990s, HMOs began to create rosters of psychologists contracted to provide service, and to place restrictions on the problems and the number of visits they would fund. Psychologists have reacted angrily to these impositions, claiming that HMOs are withholding services from individuals who need them. In 1997 psychologists, supported by their professional association, initiated a lawsuit against one of the major HMOs for wrongfully terminating them from its list of providers. They argue that such acts harm both patients and providers.[60]

While the controversy continues, it remains the case that 'There is not good evidence that the therapy as delivered in the community is effective.'[61]

Psychologists in White Coats

The re-emergence of a medical image for psychological treatment, evident in two current activities, has constituted part of the efforts to repair psychology's image.

First was the 'scramble for protection under the powerful umbrella of medicine'.[62] Psychology hoped that if it could associate itself with the strong and established profession of medicine, it could, by alliance or by default, gain the credibility it could not attain through research.

This movement has been most evident in the re-acquisition of medical concepts and terminology and in the attempt to redefine physical illnesses in emotional and psychological language.

In contrast to its earlier anti-medical stance, in the late 1970s the Psychology Industry began to remodel itself along the lines of traditional medicine. Problems became 'psychopathology' or diseases (e.g. the 'epidemic of depression'), difficulties became 'disorders' or 'syndromes', individuals again became 'patients', assessments became 'diagnoses' and outcomes were now 'prognoses'. A significant contribution to this movement was the official introduction in 1980 of the *DSM-III*, which the *American Journal of Psychiatry* described as having served to augment the 'general trend toward the remedicalization of the phenomena of psychiatry'. In an editorial in the issue discussing the *DSM-III* and psychotherapy, Chodoff concluded that 'the other purposes [beyond diagnosis] the diagnostic manual serves

[are] to provide labels for hospital, third party, and other records, and to supply data for research into the prevalence and outcome of psychiatric conditions no matter how they are treated.'[63] However, studies in the mid-1970s had shown the overall unreliability of these psychiatric labels,[64] a conclusion that was supported by Chodoff when he noted that 'treatment tends to give rise to a diagnosis'. Thus, if the *DSM* is unreliable and diagnostically imprecise, it can only be concluded that the major effect of *DSM-III* and its successors, the *DSM IV* and *IVR*, was its provision of billing codes and the consequent absorption of mental-health problems into the medical health care (and insurance) system.

Not only did psychology adopt medical terminology, it also tried to co-opt medical patients and their business, with political statements such as '60% or more of the physician visits are made by patients who demonstrate an emotional, rather than an organic, etiology for their physical symptoms.'[65]

But, rather than share their turf, psychiatrists and psychologists began fighting for the same turf. Significant in this struggle is the current trend to approach psychological problems from a biological perspective, with regard to both diagnosis and treatment. For instance, neurobiological evidence and explanations are being sought for such problems as trauma and post-traumatic stress disorder.[66] And pharmaceuticals are being tested and dispensed for the treatment not only of depressive symptoms, but also of attention deficit hyperactive disorder (e.g. Ritalin), impotence (e.g. Viagra) and alcoholism (e.g. Naltrexone).[67]

This shift towards a biological orientation has spurred the recent tactic of licensed psychologists to lobby for the right to prescribe psychoactive drugs.[68] Additionally, psychologists have attempted to be defined as 'physicians' by such regulations as the Medicare Statute or as providing 'equivalent services' to physicians.[69] Some success was achieved in this area in a 1998 decision in California to allow psychologists admitting and treatment privileges in hospitals, much like those currently held by physicians. And all this is being carried out by a profession which historically fought psychiatry, hospitalization and the use of drugs, arguing that psychotherapy was 'just as effective'.

The Customer is Always Right

The 1980s began in the United States with a period of affluence in the upper-middle-class segment of society most amenable to psychological services. The conservative, right-facing, self-serving form of Reaganomics provided the social climate for strident patriotic and tribal values, for the repression of open questioning, and for individual and national isolation and self-interest. 'A civilization [existed] in which, as never before, man [was] preoccupied with Self.'[70] The right to moral equality promoted in the 1960s was transformed by that generation, now in their forties, into a philosophy of individual achievement and acquisition, and any failure to achieve and acquire was interpreted as having a psychological cause.

As the decade progressed, the economy faltered, unemployment increased, national debts became public burdens and, for the first time in the country's history, a generation existed which anticipated a lower standard of living than its parents. People were angry at previous generations and authorities that had overspent and overused resources resulting in depletion, pollution and higher costs. It seemed as if all the present disappointments and hardships were due to what others had done in the past. People who wanted to be cured of their unhappiness and to be assured of their 'right' to wealth and success were prepared to see themselves as victims.

To borrow Cattell's words from almost a hundred years earlier, America was ripe for a new psychology. And the Psychology Industry, as always reactive to 'the noisy yammering of the secular world',[71] saw this as a business opportunity. Its response has been to refocus its attention and retool its techniques; to begin seeing people as victims of past events rather than as individuals struggling with impulses or striving to develop positive attitudes. It reinterpreted problems as the result of traumatic events rather than of negative thoughts and destructive behaviours. It defined 'regression' (going back into the past) and 'recovery' as the primary tools of the new technology.

These concepts of trauma and repression and their adaptations served to meet the needs of society and, indirectly, of the Psychology Industry. They provided a simple and saleable explanation of why people were unhappy or unsuccessful, and they placed the responsibility (the blame) outside the individual and upon others: those who generally appeared happier, wealthier or in a better life position. Through this belief, a broad new market for the Psychology Industry has been created, one that can be generalized to explain most 'problems' in life and can be easily marketed to society.

Various forms of victim-making therapies began to appear. Probably the first significant one involved the diagnosis and treatment of multiple personality disorders (MPD), later expanded and relabelled dissociative identity disorder (DID). Although as a psychological concept MPD had existed for many years, the frequency of its occurrence in its true form was considered to be rare.[72] In the 1970s, reports connecting MPD to childhood trauma began to appear in single case histories. 'Among the first and best-known was the case of Sybil, treated by Cornelia Wilbur and dramatized by Schrieber'[73] in her 1973 book *Sybil*. The *New York Times* ranked *Sybil* among the ten best-selling nonfiction books of the year and it was quickly turned into a Hollywood movie. Schrieber was deluged with letters from women thanking her for helping them understand that they were 'multiples'. It was not long before psychologists, in what Spiegel refers to as 'a whole new cult, a whole new wave of hysteria',[74] began finding cases of MPD among their patients. Quickly, psychologists began to report higher and higher frequencies, eventually claiming occurrences of one person in every hundred in the general population with much higher incidence rates in groups such as sexual-abuse survivors, hospital inpatients and chemically dependent individuals.[75] They attributed the cause to early childhood trauma, usually sexual in nature and repressed from memory. Rapidly, MPD became accepted as the explanation for many unusual or unacceptable behaviours or for the feelings of disorientation or being out of sorts (e.g. 'it's just not like me to . . .'), and as a legal defence against criminal charges.

This 'epidemic' of MPD gave rise to a host of new treatments and services which involved the acceptance of the psychologist's diagnosis[76] and the psychological 'uncovering' of trauma. In addition to providing direct service to individuals, it introduced psychologists into the legal arena in a way that had never been experienced before as clients began to report being *victims* of child abuse, sexual abuse, cult abuse and even satanic abuse. Psychology was finally gaining the exposure and status that it had been seeking, but it was gaining this in association with the legal profession rather than medicine. Whereas the medical profession had been unwilling to acknowledge the expertise of nonmedical and untrained psychologists, lawyers were eager to find 'experts' who could be employed to support their clients' cases.

But MPD was not the only victim-making technology of this retooled industry. Other formats emerged, all with an underlying framework which defined the patient as good but damaged by trauma and therefore a victim in need of the psychologist's help, and someone else as bad, a perpetrator, an enemy. Whether it was an alcoholic parent, an abusive spouse, a perverted teacher or doctor, a rude store clerk or an annoying or harassing colleague, the patient was always the innocent victim; the Other was the malevolent cause. And with the proliferation of the Psychology Industry's workforce of untrained and poorly educated technicians, the victim-making approach gained popularity. It was simple to understand and easy to sell. By aligning with the victims, accepting their reports as true and not confronting or identifying anything negative in them, victim-making psychologists achieved popularity. Not only did they explain patients' behaviours and feelings, they supported them and defended their right to retaliation and compensation in court. Psychologists appeared on television and in the media to explain social phenomena, political events and criminal behaviours. Using the *DSM* diagnoses such as post-traumatic stress disorder, they recast 'acts of God' (e.g. hurricanes and floods), acts of war (e.g. the Second World War and the conflict in and around Bosnia) and acts of foolishness as psychological events, creating victims of trauma in need of the services of the Psychology Industry.

While cartoons such as this one portrayed these 'experts' in an unflattering and disturbingly realistic light, people generally remained gullible consumers of whatever they were saying. The public listened, the courts listened and the media rarely expressed scepticism regarding even the most absurdly simplistic explanations of events. Business, it seemed, was going on as usual.

...WE NOW TURN TO AN EXPERT ON THIS SUBJECT, WHO DOESN'T ACTUALLY KNOW ANY MORE THAN WE DO. BUT HE LOOKS SINCERE, SOUNDS CONVINCING AND HAS 'DR.' IN FRONT OF HIS NAME.
NEWS
06
RAESIDE
VICTORIA TIMES-COLONIST.

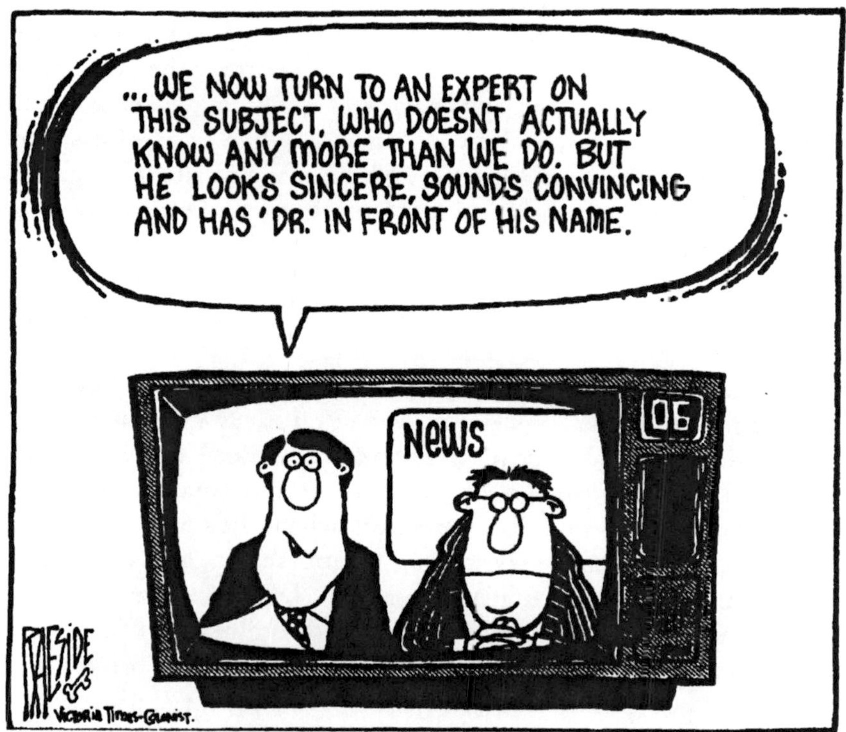

Reprinted with the permission of Adrian Raeside, 1999

Making Gidgets and Widgets: A Business Strategy

> *There seem to be rainy days ahead for psychology not because of what we have done or not done but because of major political and economic changes that seem sure to have profound effect on psychology . . . Change is in the wind, and [psychologists] have little effect on wind.*[77]

As the public image of power and expertise continued to be projected, the Psychology Industry was becoming progressively more concerned about its future in the marketplace. This note of concern was voiced, in 1994, by the chief executive of APA in relation to the 'health care reform initiatives sweeping the country, the continuing evolution of managed care, and other significant market trends affecting the practice of psychology'. Ironically, while psychologists are seeking to establish their expertise and influence in all aspects of life and promote their public prestige, many privately are struggling for their own survival.

Psychology in North America has typically relied on the health-care market, whether it has been in the formal health-care system, the private mental-health clinics or the private practices dependent on health insurance ('third party') payments. But with the failure of the Clinton health-care plan, the severe cutbacks in both the size and services of the US government and the federal funding of the Canadian system of universal health care, and the drastic reductions in individuals' discretionary monies from which they paid for therapy in the past, the future of psychology seems shaky. As Ted Morris, the treasurer of the Canadian Register of Health Service Providers in Psychology, put it, licensed 'psychologists are being excised from institutional practice faster than any other health care professional group – *we are expensive to feed and painless to drown.*'[78] Clearly, despite popular beliefs about the importance and power of psychologists and efforts by them to prove their relevance and effectiveness, they are failing to convince decision-makers and health-care administrators that they are an essential and 'valued component of mainstream health care'. 'Government spending cuts for research, health care and education have gone well beyond the fat and deep into the muscle and bone,' wrote the Canadian Psychological Association's public-affairs chair, Richard Allon. '*Our discipline is under siege.*'[79] As Morris said, when addressing his colleagues: 'Like it or not we have got *to do business differently*. This is not a false alarm but a wake up call; at issue is survival . . . I do endorse entrepreneurship and aggressive marketing . . .'[80]

Some psychologists have responded to this 'crisis' by attempting to demonstrate the cost-effectiveness of psychological insurance benefits, while others have organized to lobby public officials and launch media campaigns to gain support.[81] But at the individual level, as practitioners report that their earnings are decreasing,[82] the search for alternative ways to get paid has begun. Robert Resnick, 1995 president of the APA, put it this way: 'the way to make it when the market is changing is by diversifying, that's what corporations do. *You don't only make widgets; you make some gidgets and some widgets.*'[83]

Although some psychologists may take Resnick's advice and begin making gidgets, others, it would seem, are just relabelling their widgets. Kovacs, concerned about survival, argues, in what seems to be a glimpse of psychologizing in action, that psychologists should move out of the mental-health business and become 'consultants on life-span developmental challenges'.[84] In response, Herron and Welt commented:

> although the same type of patient problems will still be worked with . . . the names will be changed to such more palatable alternatives as 'unhappiness.' . . . [Kovacs] is, in effect, attempting to provide himself, and those who use his services, with an alternative that will be more likely to attract paying consumers . . . The approach is a marketing tool that contains economic motivation.[85]

In another attempt to redesign widgets, some psychologists have turned to defining their services as 'coaching' rather than therapy. Dr Patrick Williams, president of 'Therapist University, a virtual learning forum for therapists', markets courses on 'Building a Successful Coaching Business' and 'Learning how therapists can successfully transition into the Personal Coaching Business'.[86] In other words, at this point in the history of the Psychology Industry, the repackaging and relabelling of psychological products may be an essential component to maintaining consumer demand.

Another approach involves the use of mass-media marketing. The APA's public education campaign is a case in point, as it employs television and radio advertising, print media, a mail-out package service and a Web site encouraging visitors to 'Talk to Someone Who Can Help'. One US state, New Jersey, launched a statewide public education campaign called 'Focus on the Family' to educate the public on the availability and need for psychological services. 'Our goal is to have events statewide which bring the campaign messages to as many consumers as possible throughout the whole month of May,' Jodi Erdman, the coordinator, said.[87]

While the Psychology Industry has been effective in infusing psychology into the human experience and persuading millions of people that they suffer directly or indirectly from psychological problems, it is up to local psychologists to be innovative, entrepreneurial and aggressive; to do business differently.

In looking back over the twentieth century, one finds cause to wonder how the psychology of William James, rich with a sense of 'soul', and that of Freud and Jung with its wealth of internal life, could end up in what one psychologist called the psychological version of the fast-food industry.

In striving to secure status and position in society, psychology has surrendered its inquisitiveness and its complexity in exchange for a simplistic but more easily marketable product. In doing so it has stolen from, but tossed aside, the contextual wealth of the works of Freud and Jung, of Watson and Skinner, and of many other pioneers of the profession.

The Psychology Industry has taken the behaviouristic idea that for every effect there is a stimulus and for every problem there must be a cause outside of the person. But, discarding the behaviourists' caution about the subjectivity of looking inside the black box, it claims to know what is inside the person's mind. Calling the black box the 'unconscious', and defining the unconscious as the receptacle of traumatic memories and the continuing stimulus or cause of problems, it claims access to both the problem and the solution. The damaged child becomes the father of the dysfunctional man (or, more often, the dysfunctional woman).

It is important to note that the Psychology Industry chooses to ignore Freud's concept of the unconscious and Skinner's of operant conditioning. It refuses to acknowledge that the unconscious is far more complicated than just a mental container full of horrible memories. In so doing, it turns a blind eye to the fact that everyone constructs his or her own individual and subjective perspective on life and that 'the clinical reconstruction of early childhood experience deals with the subject's present view *about* his past, and not with the discovery of archeological artifacts that have been buried.'[88]

The Psychology Industry also disregards the behavioural principle that events have reinforcements as well as stimuli. It neglects to consider the variety of possible rewards that may foster and encourage victim-thinking and victim-acting on the part of the fabricated victim, and victim-making on the part of the psychologist. To ignore these reinforcers may be advantageous and profitable to the Psychology Industry as it maintains the person as victim, but it defeats the stated intention of psychology, which is to help people change, becoming more (rather than less) independent and functional.

If these shocking presumptions were not an actual description of the current state of the Psychology Industry, they might be laughable. But regrettably, these simplistic theories are widely applied and widely accepted in a society which naively trusts psychologists to be scientific and objective, to be optimistic and positive, and to be caring and other-oriented.

Reviewing the parallel histories in this way is not meant to imply the existence of an evil conspiracy or to suggest that psychology has been consciously designed to serve business interests and to control the minds of the public. Nor is it meant to suggest that it is inherently wrong to desire money, or to seek affluence, prestige and social status. However, as history demonstrates, psychologists have pursued their own goals at great expense to society. The psychiatrist Fuller Torrey once described psychology as 'the world's second oldest profession, remarkably similar to the first. Both involve a contract (implicit or explicit) between a specialist and a client for a service, and for this service a fee is paid.'[89] Both professions shape themselves and their services to fit the wishes and feelings of their clients, to make them feel better in body or in mind, but the underlying goal is to do whatever has to be done in order to make a living. 'Give the customer what he wants' is the motto, whether it is the pleasure of sex, the benefits of strong workers and soldiers, the thrill of self-actualization or the blamelessness of victimhood. In this liaison, American society has abandoned its moral and cultural tradition while psychology has lost its soul and neglected, even scorned, its own scientific foundation. Psychology has failed to see how it changes itself in response to the wishes and fantasies of its client. Psychologists have overlooked the influence of social and financial rewards on their own thinking and actions and failed to notice that, in pursuing their own goals, they have conformed to the common ideology, the Zeitgeist.

7

Taking Back Our Private Lives

We need to take back our private lives, to retrieve them from the intrusive interest of the market and of the social discipline (norms) so that we can live them in privacy, as diversely, eccentrically, and if the occasion demands it, as unhappily as we like.

David Smail

When the first North American edition of *Manufacturing Victims* was released in 1996, it drew volatile reactions from within the Psychology Industry. It was instantly attacked as 'a conspiracy book' and later called 'the Ripley's Believe It Or Not of Psychology', referring to the popular American newspaper cartoons which illustrate 'the odd, the unusual, and the just plain bizarre' aspects of nature which prove that truth is stranger than fiction. One psychologist, having read only a brief news report about the book, diagnosed me as suffering from 'burnout'. Another, having watched me on national television, lodged a formal complaint with my licensing board which proceeded to investigate me in the name of 'protecting the television-watching public'. It was eighteen months before the board finally dismissed the complaint, acknowledging my charter right to speak and my role as 'a social critic'.

These reactions, as well as the testimony of 'the experts' in courts and 'the healers' in their offices, are consistent with the views promoted by the Psychology Industry: that people are incapable of thinking for themselves, taking responsibility for their own actions or living their own lives. Put simply, the Psychology Industry considers and treats people as children who, regardless of age, experience, education or status must be protected, guided, sheltered, excused and disciplined.

I find the prospect of this emerging new paternalistic society in which the 'fathers' (the 'paters') are the psychologists, whose knowledge is superior and whose power is absolute, to be intolerable. So, I find myself in the role of renegade, openly challenging the authority of my profession.

Some time ago, Noam Chomsky said: 'One waits in vain for psychologists to state the limits of their knowledge.' In the summer of 1998, he added: 'I'm sure we'll continue to "wait in vain." Too many careers at stake.'[1]

Throughout this book, I have made it clear that real victims do exist and that people can truly suffer as a consequence of natural events and human cruelty. And I have pointed out that, as with anything that is real, from silk to pearls to paintings, there is always the copy, the synthetic and the counterfeit, the product made to look like the real thing. Just as there are real victims, so too are there fabricated victims, who are, by and large, the products of the current Psychology Industry, a conglomerate consisting of licensed psychologists, psychiatrists and social workers, the mental-health consultants and the vast array of lay and self-determined therapists, counsellors, helpers and healers.

Realizing this, one must face the overall harmful effects on individual lives, human relationships and civilized society, and consider what can be done to curb them. At the conclusion of the Second World War, psychology promised that, with its scientific knowledge and particular understanding of human nature, it would produce a safer and better world. However, with its technical approach to the human experience, life has become two-dimensional, black and white, good and bad; people have learned to sulk and blame. Ernest Becker realized this problem when he wrote:

> All the analysis (therapy) in the world doesn't allow the person to find out who he is and why he is here on earth. Why he has to die, and how he can make his life a triumph. It is when psychology pretends to do this, when it offers itself as a full explanation of human unhappiness, that it becomes a fraud that makes an impasse from which he cannot escape.[2]

By casting people as victims, by contending that man's inhumanity to man, as evidenced in violence and greed, can be controlled by psychological means, and that shame, unhappiness, pain, guilt and sorrow can be overcome, the Psychology Industry demonstrates a mixture of naivety and dishonesty. It robs people of their opportunities to learn from mistakes, cope with betrayal, take risks, meet obligations and comfort each other. As Bollas and Sundelson write: 'the telling aim of the health industry complex is to suppress individual freedom and to create a nation of "normopaths" or "normotics" – the abnormally normal – for whom psychological conflict is viewed at worse, as endangering or, at least, as vulgar. In the end, such anxieties reflect a fear and loathing of freedom itself.'[3]

The Psychology Industry has cast a long shadow over life in North America. And the shadow is threatening to shroud the Western world. While psychologists say 'trust me', they question and often discourage one's trust and reliance on family and friends. Instead what they offer is artificial empathy, cultivated warmth and phoney genuineness, through which they can persuade people to see life the way they see it, and live life in a psychologically ordered fashion. Years ago, psychotherapy was described as 'the purchase of friendship'. What people now need is less of this interference and more genuine relationships, which, however imperfect these may be, are reciprocal rather than purchased. As David Smail comments: 'There will no doubt always be a place for . . . kindness, encouragement and comfort, but it is surely too much to expect a professionalized, and hence interest saturated, therapy industry somehow to replace or take over the function of an ethics of human conduct.'[4]

People must learn to question the altruistic appearance of the

Psychology Industry. It is first and foremost a business, intent on selling its services and expanding its market. As such, psychologists are selling the public a bill of goods, making false promises about happiness, health and safety which they cannot fulfil.

Psychologists are in the business of posing as experts in living, claiming for themselves the ability to divine right from wrong and cause from effect. The Psychology Industry has persuaded society that the 'good life' is possible with the guidance and assistance of psychologists. It has ignored the caution of Reinhold Niebuhr that 'Goodness, armed with power is corrupted.'[5] Instead, it persists in malicious benevolence, insisting that people must live by expert advice.

These effects on individuals, relationships and social institutions constitute the most egregious harm inflicted by the Psychology Industry. They threaten the fabric of society and the principles upon which it relies. But the Psychology Industry is harmful also in other, more sweepingly pervasive ways. As Langs said: 'Therapy, as currently practiced, is neither a science nor subject to exact standards. Yet the interventions of a therapist have consequences every bit as enduring as those of a surgeon.'[6]

The Psychology Industry is not concerned, and would prefer to overlook the damage it wreaks not only on users but also on society as a whole. Most people, when they consider the work of psychologists, think of it on the level of the individual. They imagine individuals being counselled about behaviours, feelings and relationships. They believe that these people are victims who really have been abused, injured and damaged. They hear psychologists talk and testify about individual cases. What is missed entirely is the larger social effect of the industry, how the Psychology Industry is manipulating everyone to accept its victim mythology and how it is using its persuasion to enforce conformity.

Instead of freeing people to live fuller and richer lives, the Psychology Industry is creating ever more constricted and conforming ones. As Hoffer observed: 'people raised in the atmosphere of a mass movement are fashioned into incomplete and dependent human beings.'[7] David Smail adds that

> It is indeed a particular privilege of the grown-up to live a private life however he or she likes it. It is, furthermore, the business of the psychotherapist, if asked, as far as possible to help people to do precisely that, and not to try to push them into conformity with some standardized conception of 'mental health.' Rather than being, as they unwittingly too often are, representatives of a form of social discipline, psychotherapists could better become the reticent and unheroic assistants of people whose private struggles are nobody's business but their own . . .[8]

But the Psychology Industry does not accept or even acknowledge this responsibility. Instead, it allows itself to be a willing, cooperative agent of social policy, with its activities and research dependent on governmental or institutional funding. By doing so, it diminishes its capacity to step back and question the always present and unspoken assumptions that underlie the present form of society, 'an undergirding that drastically limits the universe of alternatives that social policymakers can consider'.[9] This willingness to ignore alternatives in favour of current social policies and to avoid challenging the views of policymakers is what has turned the profession into an industry. Instead of probing human nature and thereby striving to understand why the social order has come to be the way it is and how one might build a better one, psychologists have colluded to maintain the present one in which they have gained power and become part of the elite. Despite psychologists' apparent willingness to describe themselves as 'social influence purveyors', they fail to see that in assuming this role, they become pawns in a larger game of manufacturing dependent, conforming and disciplined people, the real victims of the Psychology Industry. The US Supreme Court Justice Brandeis wrote a long time ago that 'experience should teach us to be most on guard to protect liberty when the government's purposes are beneficent'; to this can be added the Psychology Industry's purposes.[10]

The closing decades of the twentieth century have seen an exponential growth in the Psychology Industry in North America and predictions have been made that there will be a further 64 per cent increase in the number of US psychologists in the next ten years,[11] leading one to worry, as Boring did, that soon 'there will be more psychologists than people in this country'. These psychologists, in the hope of furthering their own interests, have cooperated with big business, the military and government. And yet they still seem to believe that they are acting as reformers in a humanitarian sense, as they simultaneously trap millions of people in a psychological system which causes them to go backwards into the future.

With this caution in mind, what can be done?

A solution should not be expected to come from within an industry that is intent on self-protection, self-preservation and self-interest. Psychologists ignore the ethical standards they claim to uphold; 'do no harm' is a point forgotten when these professional organizations address complaints of damage from false interpreting, remembering and naming. The practice of psychologizing and victim-making is so widespread throughout the Psychology Industry that it is difficult to garner any support to stop the practice, even in its most harmful forms.

With only a few exceptions, the professional associations and licensing boards have been notably inert in carrying out their mandate to protect the public. Interestingly, the only clear warnings regarding 'recovered memory therapy' have come from psychiatric associations while the foremost psychological associations have remained silent. A report of the Royal College of Psychiatrists in the UK concludes that 'there is no evidence that recovered memory techniques can reveal memory of real events or accurately elaborate factual information about past experiences.'[12] And the Canadian Psychiatric Association released a 'position statement' cautioning its members that 'reports of recovered memories of sexual abuse may be true, but great caution should be exercised before acceptance in the absence of corroboration. Psychiatrists should be aware that excessive emphasis on recovering memories may lead to misdirection of the treatment process and unduly delay appropriate therapeutic measures.'[13] Meanwhile the psychological associations have been mute. For instance, in 1993, the APA established a working group to address the issue of memories of childhood abuse. Three years later, it submitted a report which acknowledged a split between the clinicians who believe in recovered memories, and the researchers who study human memory. It conceded that it was 'important to acknowledge frankly that we differ markedly on a wide range of issues'. And other organizations, such as the Canadian Psychological Association[14] and the British Association for Counselling,[15] have been equally equivocal in their position, making it clear that professional associations and boards can not be relied upon when issues of serious public concern conflict with those of the Psychology Industry. One possible exception is the British Psychological Society, which, while slow off the mark, is giving some indication that it has finally begun to consider the issue and to draft tentative guidelines.[16]

Recently, the APA stated that 'international psychology organizations are flourishing across the globe, giving psychologists a sea of opportunities to become involved in world affairs . . .'[17] In accepting the Award for the International Advancement of Psychology, Anthony Marsella wrote:

> The economic, political, and military dominance of Western society is rapidly spreading Western cultural lifestyles, values, and priorities across the world, creating a *Westernized global psychology*. This process can be considered a colonization of the mind. The key to the culture-change process is the power of the different parties. The West's economic, political, and military power helps make its products and lifestyles appealing. The lives of virtually all the world's citizens have been opened to Western values, lifestyles, and products through invitation, necessity, or force.
>
> For psychologists, the many global events and forces confronting people today can offer new opportunities for developing and applying their knowledge. Psychologists, as knowers and helpers, can do many things to address the problems and possibilities emerging from our global community . . . They can assist in envisioning, negotiating, designing, and evaluating a human social order and a meaningful world peace. Psychology has the opportunity to emerge as one of the most important areas of knowledge

> for the coming century – a pivotal area of inquiry and application positioned to make a difference by virtue of its expertise, values, and wisdom. Perhaps it was always an inherent part of psychology's destiny to do so.[18]

Influenced by American values and interests, this psychological imperialism is spreading around the world. To block the damaging effects of an out-of-control industry, action must be taken to stop this colonization of the mind. The American example holds important clues in this regard, which might best be understood in the context of the following story, which is said to have been Carl Jung's favourite:

> The water of life, wishing to make itself known on the face of the earth, bubbled up in an artesian well and flowed without effort or limit. People came to drink of the magic water and were nourished by it, since it was so clean and pure and invigorating. But humankind was not content to leave things in this Edenic state. Gradually they began to fence the well, charge admission, claim ownership of the property around it, make elaborate laws as to who could come to the well, put locks on the gates. Soon the well was property of the powerful and the elite. The water was angry and offended; it stopped flowing and began to bubble up in another place. The people who owned the property around the first well were so engrossed in their power systems and ownership that they did not notice that the water had vanished. They continued selling the nonexistent water, and few people noticed that the true power was gone. But some dissatisfied people searched with great courage and found the new artesian well. Soon that well was under the control of the property owners, and the same fate overtook it. The spring took itself to yet another place – and this has been going on throughout recorded history.[19]

This is a sad but essentially encouraging tale of human egotism, greed and foolishness – the defining characteristics of the Psychology

Industry. The encouragement comes not from the Psychology Industry but rather, from the central idea that, in spite of such efforts, what is most precious in human nature will somehow endure.

For the past fifty years in the United States, psychologists have been building fences, charging fees, making laws and padlocking their turf; all in an attempt to claim their role as keepers of psychological knowledge and to establish themselves as the licensed or certified dispensers of psychological wisdom and healing. Where they can, they have subverted basic truth into egocentric possessions; and where they can't, they have manufactured truths to expand their activities and to maximize their profits.

Most people assume that licensing exists to protect the public but, in fact, it serves to protect only that privileged group in society who possess the credentials. Shortly before his death, Rollo May reflected on the early days of licensing. He described the time in the mid-1950s, the 'dangerous years' when the American Medical Association threatened to outlaw nonmedical psychotherapists and to take ownership of psychotherapy. For years May lived in intense anxiety that his practice would be outlawed. Eventually, he and his colleagues concluded that 'the best step for us as psychologists would be to clarify all the different branches of psychotherapy' and they organized a conference on the training, practice and safeguards of psychotherapy. 'From that moment on, the fact that psychotherapy was conducted by psychologists . . . was then accepted in the various legislatures around the country.' May went on to describe a conversation he had at that time with Carl Rogers:

> expecting his enthusiastic help, I was taken aback by his stating that he was not sure whether it would be good or not to have psychologists licensed . . . During the following years, I kept thinking of Carl Rogers' doubts about our campaign for licensing. I think he foresaw that we psychologists could be as rigid as any other group, and this certainly has been demonstrated . . .[20]

Rogers's hesitation should have been heeded; licensing should never have happened. Instead of resisting the threat, psychologists took on the very nature of those that threatened them. They claimed joint ownership of psychotherapy, only extending the menacing monopoly to include them. And they licensed themselves to appear similar to those medical doctors that had earlier threatened their existence. They became rigid and controlling, deriving their identity from their licences, titles and credentials. They used these licences to give themselves the authority to decide who and what is normal and abnormal, good and bad, healthy and sick. And other groups, seeing how well this strategy worked, followed suit and established their own self-regulating licensing boards, all of which have served the hidden goals of self-promotion rather than the stated aims of protecting the public.

It is these symbols of authority, the licences and credentials, totems of arrogance, that must be banned or eliminated in order for society to survive. It is only in removing these vestments of power and influence that society will be able to take back its right to psychological freedom, where people are accepted or judged by their families, friends and peers, and not by self-ordained experts.

While eliminating licensing would be a crucial step, it is clearly only one of several which need to be taken. Throughout history there have always been seers, astrologers, healers, alchemists, diviners and advisers who offered their services to the eager, the desperate and the gullible true believers. It would be naive to expect that psychologists would suddenly disappear. They will undoubtedly continue to exist and practise with or without their licences, finding customers for their various brands of snake oil.

Other steps which should be taken include:

- **Stop or avoid insurance coverage for psychological services.**

In North America, third-party payments have allowed many fabricated victims unlimited access to psychological services and provided the Psychology Industry with a major source of income.

All indications are that, to date, all insurance-funded systems have lost money for insurers, provoking the current shift towards managed care in the United States which limits the number of sessions, creates indices which relate diagnoses to treatment method and number of sessions, and opens psychological services to competitive bidding. While these new measures will shorten the free ride, they may have a paradoxical effect. To compensate for the reduced income per client, the Psychology Industry may very well work to increase the variety of victims, each having the possibility of receiving treatment funding from alternative sources such as those provided through the courts, businesses and professional liability insurers.

In the United States, some moves are already afoot to support only established treatments that address immediate problems without dwelling on the aetiology or imaginary causes.[21] Recently a number of psychologists wrote to the US Congress suggesting that all relevant sections of health-care codes specify that:

> No tax or tax exempt monies may be used for any form of health care treatment, including any form of psychotherapy, that has not been proven safe and effective by rigorous, valid and reliable scientific investigation and accepted as safe and effective by a substantial majority of the relevant scientific community.[22]

Although this may be a step forward, the Psychology Industry should not be allowed to oversee this activity, given its abysmal track record in self-regulation, for it would enjoy a clear benefit in approving techniques based on limited or flawed research. There is the danger that the establishment of 'validated therapies' could end up spawning a new sub-industry as demonstrated by the number of manuals and workshops that have begun to appear promoting 'proven' therapies.

• Stop the public sanctioning of the Psychology Industry.

There is a serious need to challenge the pervasive and expensive sanctioning of psychological services through such things as victim support and counselling, court-ordered treatment, mandated treatment for addictions and work-performance problems, and compensation for psychological stress and damage.

In an effort to appear humane, courts have moved towards referring for psychological treatment not only crime victims but also those who have been convicted of a crime in which 'psychological problems' were a factor. In some jurisdictions, employers are also being mandated to provide treatment for employees with psychological problems, such as alcohol and substance abuse or sexual disorders. Similarly, workers' compensation programmes now include provisions for job-related stress, and stress debriefings are required for both victims of trauma and emergency personnel. While these treatments generally lack any proof of their long-term effectiveness, they have become legally sanctioned, publicly endorsed and accepted, and are widely used. Susan Sarnoff, in referring to publicly accredited psychological services as 'sanctified snake oil', states that government support and funding of 'junk social science' creates an implied approval of these bogus methods that is unwarranted and wasteful of tax dollars. She warns that what is truly dangerous, at this time in history, is not that 'snake oil' is for sale but rather that it is legitimized by these official stamps of approval.[23]

• Stop psychologists from influencing the Justice System.

Bogus psychology experts, often supported by their professional organizations, mislead the courts daily, deluding judges and juries into believing that their procedures and opinions are uncontroversial and based on responsible, scientific research. In fact, this activity has become so rampant that the proposed Truth and Responsibility in

Mental Health Practices Act requires 'all psychotherapists and social scientists to *tell the truth* in American courts of law.'[24] One can only hold in contempt a profession in which honesty must be legally mandated when all other citizens voluntarily accept this as their ethical and legal responsibility.

Junk psychology is a serious threat to the integrity of the legal system, and, with irresponsible testimony by psychologists reaching epidemic proportion in some jurisdictions, the only solution is to disallow any involvement of psychologists posing as experts. This would remove the status which allows beliefs, opinions and myths to be expressed as 'facts' and 'professional knowledge'; it would allow the judicial system to recover from psychological contamination.

- **Demand truth in advertising.**

Like others whose products and services are sold in the marketplace, psychologists should be required to substantiate their claims of knowledge and effectiveness. While the public continues to be swayed by an aura of honesty and infallibility and presumes that psychologists not only know the truth but also speak it, such is neither the case nor even a professional requirement.

Whether privately in therapy sessions, or publicly in advertisements, seminars and statements to the media, psychologists must be held accountable for their claims and prevented from misleading the public. They should be reported to their associations and licensing boards, which should be pressured to take action. And if these professional organizations continue to sanction such activity, they should be reported to the advertising councils and to consumer-protection groups, and exposed in the media. The image of professionalism should not be allowed to protect the Psychology Industry from the laws and regulations applied to other commercial operations. Society deserves the same protection from consumer fraud and product harm with psychological services as it is entitled to from the auto or appliance industries.

• Hold psychologists legally responsible for their activities.

The current controversy regarding recovered memories is evidence that the Psychology Industry can *use* patients in social causes that are based on popularized opinions. Some have even made 'social action' a recognized part of treatment.[25] For instance, Laura Brown, an APA presidential candidate in 1997, writes that her psychological practice with clients has a social-justice orientation which includes 'subverting patriarchy in [her] office, on the witness stand, and in the classroom'.[26]

What is needed is to reaffirm psychologists' responsibility and liability for what they do, and to curtail their larger goals as social influencers. Psychologists need to be held accountable for the therapy methods they use and, if these methods are controversial or unproven, they must be identified as such at the outset, with all clients being warned of the risk of potential harm and the significant possibility that interpretations and memories will be inaccurate. In addition, they deserve to be made aware of the psychologist's stance regarding social and legal actions. Both society and the courts understand the role of accomplice, and such a concept must be applied to therapists involved in malicious or wrongful accusations and actions. The British law lords have opened the way for people wrongly accused of crimes – including men falsely accused of rape – to sue their accusers for damages. One of the judges, Lord Keith, stated: 'To deny any remedy to a person whose liberty has been interfered with as a result of unfounded and malicious accusations . . . would constitute a serious denial of justice.'[27]

Similar legal sentiment in the United States has led to a growing number of civil suits against psychologists, holding them responsible for their actions. In 1995 a psychiatrist, Dr Diane Humenansky, was sued by two former patients for, among other things, the creation of false memories. The juries awarded them $2.6 million and $2.5 million; at that time 'the two largest amounts ever awarded from a psychiatrist on trial'.[28] Two 1998 settlements on comparable grounds resulted in awards of $5.8 million and $10.4 million.

• Redirect the funding of ineffective psychological treatment programmes so as to address pressing social needs.

In the early 1980s, Zilbergeld wrote: 'millions of people today seek therapy for personal and interpersonal discomforts that less affluent societies would regard as trivial.'[29] Society can no longer afford such luxuries. Psychological programmes are, by and large, an extravagant distraction from the real problems that affect people's wellbeing. They are the pseudo-treatments that contribute to the income of the Psychology Industry, while doing little to treat society's ills. Meanwhile, the more significant issues of poverty, nutrition, employment, medical care, education and even law enforcement are negatively affected as society's attention and resources get diverted to trivialized versions of violence and the self-indulgent whining of those already better off.

Rather than hire psychologists to go into the schools to teach self-esteem, teach the students skills with which they can build self-respect. Rather than employ psychologists to teach the current version of parenting, provide food, housing and parenting relief to poor families. Rather than make biopolitical knee-jerk responses to violence, challenge the Psychology Industry's exaggerated definition of violence, and put the focus back on efforts to deal with real crime. Rather than send trauma counsellors to disaster sites, apply the funds to meet the immediate social and economic needs of those affected. Rather than promote expensive demands for treatment for illusive mental-health problems, attend to the needs of the seriously mentally ill who have been abandoned in the streets and alleys.[30]

For society, the real danger to be found in the Psychology Industry is not in false memories or false allegations. It is in the false thinking and false living which are its primary effects. The Psychology Industry may abandon long-term therapy for shorter forms, more likely to be insured. It may discard recovered-memory therapy in much the same way that a large corporation jettisons a subsidiary that either loses money or causes internal problems. But society must not be fooled by these actions.

Whether in recovered-memory therapy or short-term cognitive therapy, psychologists seek to impose their view of how people should think, feel and act, generally ignoring the implications of their opinions and coercive techniques, and the conformity and mediocrity that they are imposing. The ancient Delphic injunction to 'Know thyself' referred neither to memories of the past nor to a psychologically healthy self-image. It required that individuals know their character, their strengths and limitations, their needs and gifts, their desire for truth and their tendency to avoid it. But it is deception and self-deception, rather than these aspects of self-knowledge, that the Psychology Industry fosters.

Most psychologists, if they looked back a hundred years, would hold Galton's theory about intelligence and eugenics with disdain, yet they fail to recognize the same kind of rigidity and egocentrism in their own theories. They go about their work seemingly unaware that their own self-interests and privileged social positions have more influence on their thoughts and actions than their research does. They have pursued and achieved social influence and economic gain, remaining blind to the fact that, in doing so, they have become pawns of institutions, industries and governments. Psychology has abdicated its fundamental intellectual and moral responsibility for simple honesty, intellectual autonomy, critical self-scrutiny and humane respect. Instead it promotes cognitive distortions, self-aggrandizement and social prejudice.

To stop this, it will be necessary to recognize that the well has run dry, that the power has gone, that the practice and profession of psychology is bankrupt. It does not have enough assets and resources to meet its obligations. If people take back their basic right to think for themselves, to exercise their common sense in finding solutions to their own problems, they can stop falling prey to the fantasies of professional experts. Society can then begin to reacquire the human traits of tolerance, understanding and compassion.

Some colleagues have suggested that such an aggressive stance against the Psychology Industry may result in throwing the baby out with the bathwater. But if psychologists continue to market their wares in such unethical ways, I think that this 'baby' that I am accused of throwing away will be killed anyway; that is, of course, assuming that there is a baby to be found in this murky water.

There is too much wrong with psychology; with its actions, institutions and professional organizations. Those within the Psychology Industry, as well as those outside, have cautioned it, criticized it, warned it; and yet it remains unchanged, going about business in its customary way. It can neither reform itself from within nor should it be allowed to try. It should be stopped from doing what it is doing to people. And while the Psychology Industry is being dismantled, people can boycott psychological products and services, protest the influence of the Psychology Industry and resist being manufactured into victims. And they can wonder what would happen if philosophy took back the issues of 'soul' (psyche) and 'meaning', science took back the study of the body and behaviour, friendship took back its place as the source of consolation and encouragement, and everyone, fabricated victims included, took back their own private lives.

Afterword

Many readers of the North American editions of *Manufacturing Victims* have contacted me to let me know how the book was useful to them in raising questions, challenging 'experts', making arguments, winning legal cases and facing moral dilemmas. I trust that this UK edition will also prove to contain useful information. And it is my hope that this information will be used by sensible people in their own efforts to purge the legal system, health care, education, religion and their own personal lives of the harmful influence emanating from the Psychology Industry.

Readers are invited to visit the book's frequently updated Web site at: http://scholefieldhouse.com/mv/

I am pleased to respond to comments, reactions, questions or criticisms sent by e-mail (td@scholefieldhouse.com) or in letters mailed to my publisher.

Tana Dineen
Victoria, B.C., Canada
March 1999

Notes

Foreword

1 See Illich, Ivan. *Limits to Medicine. Medical Nemesis – the Expropriation of Health.* London: Marion Boyars, 1976.

Introduction

1 Dineen, Tana. 'Diagnostic Decision Making in Psychiatry'. Unpublished doctoral thesis, University of Saskatchewan, Saskatoon, 1975.
2 See *Smiling Through Tears* by Pamela Freyd and Eleanor Goldstein. (Boca Raton, FL: Upton Books, 1997.)
3 Herman, Judith Lewis. *Trauma and Recovery.* New York: Basic Books, 1992. pp. 134–35.
4 'Responding to Oklahoma City's needs.' *APA Monitor.* Washington, DC: American Psychological Association, June 1995.
5 West, Lola, et al. 'Operation Desert Storm: The response of a social work outreach team.' *Work in Health Care,* 1993, 19(2). pp. 81–98.
6 'Women's safety illusory when males turn violent.' *APA Monitor,* February 1994.
7 'McBain conference a major success.' *Rapport,* 2, April 1994.
8 'Abuse widespread, researchers show.' *APA Monitor,* February 1994. p. 17.
9 Dorfman, Rachelle A., et al. 'Screening for depression among a well elderly population.' *Social Work,* 40(3), May 1995.
10 'Pamela's PhD in fame.' *Daily Telegraph* (London), 12 December 1995. p. 17.

11 VandenBos, Gary R., Cummings, Nicholas A., and DeLeon, Patrick H. 'A century of psychotherapy: Economic and environmental influences.' In *The History of Psychotherapy: A Century of Change.* Freedheim, Donald K. (ed.), Washington, DC: American Psychological Association, 1992.
12 1995 phone survey reported in the *APA Monitor,* June 1995; Kalellin, Peter. *Pick Up Your Couch and Walk!* New York: Crossroad, 1993.
13 Schaef, Anne Wilson. *Beyond Therapy, Beyond Science.* San Francisco: Harper, 1992.
14 Fischer, A. 'Der praktische Psychologe – ein neuer Beruf.' *Der Kunstwart and Kulturwart,* 1913, 26, p. 313. Cited in Geuter, Ulfried. *The Professionalization of Psychology in Nazi Germany.* London: Cambridge University Press, 1992.
15 Henry, William E., Sims, John H., and Spray, S. Lee. *The Fifth Profession: Becoming a Psychotherapist.* San Francisco: Jossey Bass Behavioral Science Series, 1971.
16 Fox, Ronald E. (past president of the APA) 'Training professional psychologists for the twenty-first century.' *American Psychologist,* 49(3), 1994.
17 Sam Keen, former editor of *Psychology Today.* Personal communication, 1993.
18 Sykes, Charles. *A Nation of Victims: The Decay of the American Society.* New York: St Martin's Press, 1992.
19 'Haunting memories of a war a lifetime ago' by Mitchell Landsberg of the Associated Press (Montrose, NY), 13 August 1995.
20 Bard, Morton, and Sangrey, Dawn. *The Crime Victim's Book.* New York: Basic Books, 1979.

Chapter 1

1 'Not for the timid: Details of sex assaults show true savagery.' *Vancouver Sun,* 27 March 1993. pp. B10–11.
2 From Robert McAfee Brown's preface (p. vi) to the 1986 Bantam edition of *Night* which was first published in 1960.
3 Wiesel, Elie. *Night.* New York: Bantam Books, 1960. pp. 72–73.
4 Ibid. p. 106.
5 Szasz, Thomas. *The Myth of Psychotherapy: Mental Healing as Religion, Rhetoric, and Repression.* Garden City, NY: Anchor Press/Doubleday, 1978. p. 205.
6 Gross, Martin L. *The Psychological Society: The Impact – and the Failure – of Psychiatry, Psychotherapy, Psychoanalysis and the Psychological Revolution.* New York: Random House, 1978.

7 Herman, Judith. *Trauma and Recovery.* New York: Basic Books, 1992. p. 1. (Italics added.)

8 In a letter from William James to Theodore Fournoy, dated 28 September 1909. (Italics added.)

9 Lifton, Robert Jay. *Death in Life: Survivors of Hiroshima.* New York: Random House, 1967. p. 1. (Italics added.)

10 Lifton, Robert Jay. *The Broken Connection: On Death and the Continuity of Life.* New York: Simon & Schuster, 1979. p. 179. (Italics added.)

11 Lifton. *The Broken Connection.* p. 3. (Italics added.)

12 Ibid. p. 491.

13 Wiesel, Elie. *From the Kingdom of Memory: Reminiscences.* New York: Summit Books, 1990. pp. 120–21.

14 Lifton. *Death in Life.* p. 36.

15 Ibid. p. 10. (Italics added.)

16 Lifton. *The Broken Connection.* p. 169.

17 Kubler-Ross, Elisabeth. *On Death and Dying: What the Dying Have to Teach Doctors, Nurses, Clergy and Their Own Families.* New York: Collier Books, Macmillan, 1969.

18 Frankl, Victor E. *The Unheard Cry for Meaning.* New York: Simon & Schuster, 1978. p.87.

19 'Not for public consumption.' *Vancouver Sun*, 29 May 1993.

20 Wiesel. *From the Kingdom of Memory.* pp. 170–71. (Italics added.)

21 Hoppe, Klaus D. 'The psychodynamics of concentration camp victims.' *The Psychoanalytic Forum*, 1(1), 1966, pp. 76–85. Cited by Des Pres in *The Survivor.* p. 155. (Italics added.)

22 Des Pres, Terrence. *The Survivor.* New York: Oxford University Press, 1976. p. 155.

23 Bettelheim, Bruno. *Surviving and Other Essays.* New York: Vintage Books/ Random House, 1980. pp. 24–25. (Italics added.)

24 Bettelheim's paper entitled 'Individual and mass behaviour in extreme situations' was turned down many times before being published in the *Journal of Abnormal and Social Psychology*, Vol. 38 (October 1943), pp. 417–52.

25 Bettelheim. *Surviving.* p. 36.

26 Bettelheim, Bruno. *The Informed Heart: Autonomy in a Mass Age.* New York: Free Press, 1960. p. 114.

27 Bettelheim. *Surviving.* pp. 28–35. (Italics added.)

28 Des Pres. *The Survivor.* p. 158.

29 Bettelheim. *The Informed Heart.* pp. 111–12 and 116. (Italics added.)

30 Ibid. p. 131.

31 Ibid. p. 231.
32 Bettelheim. *Surviving*. p. 35.
33 Bettelheim. *The Informed Heart*. p. 131.
34 Pollak, Richard. *The Creation of Dr B.: A Biography of Bruno Bettelheim*. New York: Simon & Schuster, 1996.
35 Lehman-Haupt, Christopher. 'Psychologist an "empty fortress" in unsparing new biography.' *New York Times* (reprinted in the Toronto *Globe and Mail*, 18 January 1997).
36 A section title in *Aftershock: Surviving the Delayed Effects of Trauma, Crisis and Loss* by Andrew E. Slaby (New York: Villard Books, 1989).
37 Segal, Julius. *Winning Life's Toughest Battles*. New York: McGraw-Hill Books, 1986. (Italics added.)
38 Lifton. *Death in Life*. pp. 491–92.
39 Bard, Morton, and Sangrey, Don. *The Crime Victim's Book*. New York: Basic Books, 1979. pp. 10, 76.
40 Des Pres. *The Survivor*. p. 157.
41 Segal. *Winning Life's Toughest Battles*. p. 2.
42 Bettelheim. *The Informed Heart*. p. 251.
43 Segal. *Winning Life's Toughest Battles*. p. 2. (Italics added.)
44 Ibid. pp. 2–3.
45 Weinfeld, M., Sigal, J. J., and Eaton, W. W. 'Long-term effects of the holocaust on selected social attitudes and behaviours of survivors: A cautionary note.' *Social Forces*, 60, September 1981, pp. 1–19.
46 This study by Antonovsky, Moaz, Dowty, and Wijsnbeek (1971) was cited by Des Pres in *The Survivor*. See also Antonovsky, Anton. *Health, Stress, and Coping*. New York: Jossey-Bass, 1979.
47 Suedfeld, Peter. 'Homo invictus: The indomitable species.' *Canadian Psychology*, 38(3), 1997, pp. 164–73.
48 Rothchild, Sylvia (ed.) *Voices from the Holocaust*. New York: New American Library, 1981. p. 7.
49 Ibid. p. 313.
50 Garmezy, Norman. 'Forward.' In Werner, E., and Smith, R. S. *Vulnerable but Invincible*. New York: McGraw-Hill, 1982, pp. xiii–xix.

Chapter 2

1 Des Pres, Terrence. *The Survivor.* New York: Oxford University Press, 1976. p. 13.
2 Hayes, Nelson. *Adult Children of Alcoholics Remember.* New York: Ballantine, 1989. pp. 242–43.
3 Sykes, Charles J. *A Nation of Victims: The Decay of the American Character.* New York: St Martin's Press. 1992. p. 18.
4 Gondolf, Lynn. In 'Doors of Memory' by Ethan Watters, *Mother Jones,* January 1993. p. 26.
5 Carroll, Lewis. *Through the Looking Glass.*
6 Beyerstein, Barry L. 'Why bogus therapies seem to work.' *Skeptical Inquirer,* Sept/Oct 1997. pp. 29–42.
7 Marie, Jan. '31 symptoms of physical, emotional, and sexual trauma.' Cited by Susan F. Smith, 'Body memories: And other pseudo-scientific notions of "survivor psychology."' *Issues in Child Abuse Accusations,* 5(4), 1993. pp. 22–234.
8 Fiore, Edith. *You Have Been Here Before: A Psychologist Looks at Past Lives.* New York: Ballantine Books, 1978. pp. 6–7.
9 Williams, M. H. 'The bait-and-switch tactic in psychotherapy.' *Psychotherapy,* 22, 1985, 110–13. p. 111.
10 Schaef, Anne W. *Beyond Therapy, Beyond Science: A New Model for Healing the Whole Person.* San Francisco: Harper San Francisco, 1992. p. 94.
11 Bass, Ellen, and Davis, Laura. *The Courage to Heal: A Guide for Women Survivors of Child Sexual Abuse.* New York: Harper & Row (3rd revised ed. Harper Perennial, 1994). pp. 24, 37.
12 Pittman, Frank, III. 'A buyer's guide to psychotherapy.' *Psychology Today,* Jan/Feb 1994. pp. 52–53.
13 Slaby, Andrew E. *Aftershock: Surviving the Delayed Effects of Trauma, Crisis and Loss.* New York: Villard Books, 1989. pp. 4–5.
14 Blume, Sue E. *Secret Survivors: Uncovering Incest and Its Aftereffects in Women.* New York: John Wiley, 1989. pp. xiii, 5.
15 Feinberg, Mortimer R., Feinberg, Gloria, and Tarrant, John J. *Leavetaking.* New York: Simon & Schuster, 1978. pp. 9–12.
16 Pasley, Laura. 'Misplaced Trust.' *Skeptical Inquirer,* 1994. p. 65.
17 Fiore, Edith. *You Have Been Here Before.* pp. 5–6.
18 From an interview on the television programme 'The Fifth Estate'. Cited

in Ofshe, Richard, and Watters, Ethan. *Making Monsters: False Memories, Psychotherapy, and Sexual Hysteria.* New York: Charles Scribner's Sons, 1994. p. 223.

19 Gondlof, Lynn. Cited in *Survivor Psychology: The Dark Side of a Mental Health Mission* by Susan Smith. Boca Raton, FL: Upton Books, 1995. p. 22.

20 Statement made by Richard Ofshe on the Dennis Prager American TV show, June 1995.

21 Attributed to APA's past president Ronald Fox in 'Fox identifies top threats to professional psychology' by Sara Martin, *APA Monitor*, March 1995. p. 44.

22 Herman. *Trauma and Recovery*. p. 177.

23 Miller, Alice. *Banished Knowledge*. New York: Doubleday, 1990. pp. 2, 4.

24 Spiegel, H. 'Hypnosis and evidence: Help or hindrance?' *Annals of the New York Academy of Science*, 1980, 347. p. 78.

25 Fiore. *You Have Been Here Before*. p. 6.

26 Cote, Isabelle. 'Adult recollections of childhood trauma.' A paper presented to the 74th annual meeting of the Ontario Psychiatric Association, Toronto, January 1994. p. 15.

27 *Michelle Remembers*, co-authored by Michelle Smith and her psychiatrist husband Lawrence Pazder (New York: Congdon & Lattes, 1980), was the first satanic-cult survivor story to become a bestseller.

28 Robert Kelly, the owner of the Little Rascals daycare in Edenton, North Carolina, was convicted in 1993 of sexually abusing twelve children and sentenced to twelve consecutive life terms. Dawn Wilson, the centre's cook, was also convicted and sentenced to a life term. In May 1995 these convictions were overturned by the state Court of Appeals. Similar cases have been reported in the popular media (see 'The Demons of Edenton' in *Elle*, November 1993, pp. 139–42, and 'Unspeakable acts' in *Good Housekeeping*, October 1995, p. 204) and discussed in academic books (Cecil, Stephen J., and Bruck, Maggie, *Jeopardy in the Courtroom: A Scientific Analysis of Children's Testimony*. Washington, DC: American Psychological Association, 1995.)

29 Interview with Harold Levy, 3 November 1995.

30 Interview with Alan Gold, 7 November 1995.

31 Herman. *Trauma and Recovery*. p. 158.

32 Frank, J. D., and Frank, J. B. *Persuasion and Healing: A Comparative Study of Psychotherapy*. (3rd edn) Baltimore: Johns Hopkins University Press, 1991. pp. 8–9.

33 Kleinman, A. *Rethinking Psychiatry: From Cultural Category to Personal Experience*. New York: Free Press, 1988.

34 Frank and Frank. *Persuasion and Healing*. p. 9.

35 Schofield, W. *Psychotherapy: The Purchase of Friendship*. Englewood Cliffs, NJ: Spectrum Books, Prentice-Hall, 1964. p. 27.
36 Jasper, K. *The Nature of Psychotherapy: A Critical Appraisal.* J. Hoenig and M. W. Hamilton (trans.) Chicago: Phoenix Books, University of Chicago Press, 1964. p. 8.
37 Peele, Stanton. *Diseasing of America: Addiction Treatment Out of Control.* Lexington, Mass.: Lexington Books, 1989. p. 49. (Citing R. Longabaugh, 'Evaluating recovery out-comes', presented at a conference, Program on Alcohol Issues, University of California, San Diego, 4–6 February 1988.)
38 American Psychiatric Association. *Diagnostic and Statistical Manual (DSM-IV).* Washington, DC: American Psychiatric Association, 1994.
39 Showalter, Elaine. *Hystories: Hysterical Epidemics and Modern Media.* New York: Columbia University Press, 1997. p. 17.
40 Peebles, Mary Jo. *Posttraumatic Stress Disorder: A historical perspective on diagnosis and treatment.* Topeka, KS: Menninger Foundation, 1989. pp. 274–86.
41 Scrignar, C. B. *Post Traumatic Stress Disorder: Diagnosis, Treatment and Legal Issues.* Westport, Conn.: Praeger, 1984. p. 2.
42 'There is a war between the sexes. Rape victims, battered women, and sexually abused children are its casualties.' Herman. *Trauma and Recovery*. p. 32.
43 'Cardinal Hume urges killer to give himself up to police.' *The Times* (London), 12 December 1995. p. 5.
44 'Pupils who saw murder "face years of trauma".' *Evening Standard* (London), 11 December 1995. p. 6.
45 Dantzer, Robert. *The Psychosomatic Delusion: Why the Mind Is Not the Source of All Our Ills.* New York: Free Press, 1993. p. i.
46 Eliot, Robert S. *From Stress to Strength.* New York: Bantam Books, 1994. p. 6.
47 Williams, Redford, and Williams, Virginia. *Anger Kills.* New York: Random House, 1993. p. xii.
48 Elliott, Glen. 'Stress and Illness'. In Stanley Cheron (ed.) *Psychosomatic Medicine: Theory, Physiology and Practice*, Vol. 1. Madison, Conn.: International Universities Press, 1989. pp. 45–90.
49 Pack Stroup, Heather, and Herndon, Paul L. 'Asserting a greater role towards health: expanding visions of psychology practice.' *Practitioner*, Vol. 8, 1, February 1995. p. 22.
50 Bruce Charash in his book *Heart Myths* (New York: Viking Press, 1991) listed the cardiac-prone personality as a popular myth.
51 Simonton, O. Carl, Matthews-Simonton, Stephanie, and Creighton, James L. *Getting Well Again: The New Best-Seller About the Simontons' Revolutionary*

Life-Saving Self-Awareness Techniques. New York: Bantam Books, 1981.

52 Simonton et al. *Getting Well Again*. p. 105.

53 *R. v. Size*, Toronto, Canada; the judge's report was released on 27 February 1991.

54 Kanin, Eugene, J. 'False Rape Allegations.' *Archives of Sexual Behavior*, 23(1), 1994.

55 'Raging Bulls: Tom and Roseanne' was a feature story in *People* magazine, 2 May 1994. pp. 34–58. Roseanne's retraction of the charges, made in late April, was reported in news services across America (e.g. *Times-Colonist*, 26 April 1994).

56 Roiphe, Katie. *The Morning After: Sex, Fear and Feminism on Campus*. Boston: Little, Brown, 1993. pp. 39–41.

57 'Stress Sex' by Carol Lynn Mithers was in the September 1993 issue of *Ladies' Home Journal*. pp. 62–72.

58 'Stress pileup can lead to murder, say experts.' *Associated Press* (Union, South Carolina), 5 November 1994.

59 Glenys Kaufman-Kantor of the Family Research Lab at the University of New Hampshire, cited in 'Stress pileup can lead to murder, say experts.'

60 Although Bianchi did not admit to posing as a counterfeit victim, the evidence that he did so was compelling. See O'Brien, Darcy. *Two of a Kind: The Hillside Stranglers*. New York: New American Library, 1985.

61 Orne, Martin T., Dinges, David F., and Orne, Emily Carota. 'On the differential diagnosis of multiple personality in the forensic context.' *International Journal of Clinical and Experimental Hypnosis*, 1984, XXXII(2). pp. 118–69.

62 See Feldman, Marc D., Ford, Charles V., and Reinhold, Toni. *Patient or Pretender*. New York: John Wiley, 1985. p. 274.

63 *For the Sake of the Children: Report of the Special Joint Committee on Child Custody and Access*. December 1998. Canadian Publications Services, Ottawa.

64 APA at http://www.apa.org/pubinfo/harass.html (In researching this book, the author challenged the data and the site subsequently was closed pending revision.)

65 For more information: http://pw2.netcom.com/~schorrig/psych.html

66 In 1994, a psychologist was found guilty of misconduct, suspended from practising, and ordered to attend specified courses to increase his sensitivity to patients who reported sexual abuse. The primary allegation was that he had confronted a patient on the possibility that she was attempting to use her 'sexual abuse to scam the insurance at work'. (Disciplinary hearing in the *Bulletin of the College of Psychologists of Ontario*, Vol. 21, No. 2, November 1994. pp. 7–9.)

67 Kottler, Jeffrey A. *The Compleat Therapist.* San Francisco: Jossey-Bass, 1991. p. 12.
68 Sykes. *A Nation of Victims.* p. 18.

Chapter 3

1 William James. 'A plea for psychology as a natural science.' (1892) in *Collected Essays and Reviews* (1920).
2 Revel, Jean-François. *The Flight from Truth.* New York: Random House, 1991. p. 18.
3 The National Surgical Adjuvant Breast and Bowel Project at the University of Pittsburgh.
4 Canadian Press, 21 September 1994.
5 Burt, C. 'Ability and income.' *British Journal of Educational Psychology*, 13, 1943. p. 200.
6 Eysenck, H. J., and Kamin, Leon. *The Intelligence Controversy.* New York: John Wiley, 1981. p. 98.
7 Hearnshaw, L. S. *Cyril Burt: Psychologist.* Ithaca, NY: Cornell University Press, 1979. Joynson, R. B. *The Burt Affair.* London: Routledge, 1989. Fletcher, R. 'Intelligence, equality, character, and education.' *Intelligence*, 15, 1991. pp. 139–49.
8 *Changing the Landscape: Ending Violence – Achieving Equality, Final Report of the Canadian Panel on Violence Against Women*, Statistics Canada, November 1993. Women's Safety Project first appeared as Appendix A of *Changing the Landscape.*
9 Fekete, John. *Moral Panic: Biopolitics Rising.* Montreal: Robert Davies, 1994.
10 Gilbert, Neil. 'The phantom epidemic of sexual assault.' *The Public Interest*, 103, 1991. p. 63.
11 Italics added for emphasis.
12 See Koss, Mary, Gidycz, Christine A., and Wisniewski, Nadine. 'The scope of rape: Incidence and prevalence of sexual aggression and victimization in a national sample of higher education students.' *Journal of Consulting and Clinical Psychology*, 55(2), 1987. pp. 162–70.
13 Marone, Nicky. *Women and Risk: How to Master Your Fears and Do What You Never Thought You Could Do.* New York: St Martin's Press, 1992.
14 Peterson, Christopher, Maier, Seteven F., and Seligman, Martin E. P. *Learned Helplessness: A Theory for the Age of Personal Control.* New York: Oxford University Press, 1993. p. 233.

15 Marone. *Women and Risk*. p. xi. (Italics added.)
16 Peterson et al. *Learned Helplessness*. p. 16.
17 Huber, Peter. *Galileo's Revenge: Junk Science in the Courtroom*. New York: HarperCollins, 1991. p. 32.
18 Smail, David. *Taking Care: An Alternative to Therapy*. London: J. M. Dent & Sons, 1987. p. 80.
19 Nemiah, John C. 'Classical Psychoanalysis.' In *American Handbook of Psychiatry: Volume Five – Treatment*. (2nd edn.) Daniel X. Freedman and Jarl E. Dyrud (eds.) New York: Basic Books, pp. 163–82.
20 Hamburg, David A., et al. 'Report of Ad Hoc Committee on Central Fact-Gathering Data of the American Psychoanalytic Association,' *Journal of the American Psychoanalytic Association*, October 1967, pp. 841–61.
21 Ackner, Lois F. *How to Survive the Loss of a Parent*. New York: William Morrow & Co., 1993. p. 209.
22 Zilbergeld, Bernie. *The Shrinking of America: Myths of Psychological Change*. Boston: Little, Brown & Co., 1983. p. 118.
23 M. B. Parloff, 'Can psychotherapy research guide the policy maker?' *American Psychologist*, 34, 1979. pp. 296–306.
24 Eysenck, Hans J. 'The effects of psychotherapy: An evaluation.' *Journal of Consulting Psychology*, 16, 1952. pp. 319–24.
25 Eysenck, Hans J. 'The effects of psychotherapy.' *International Journal of Psychiatry*, 1, 1965. pp. 97–168.
26 Kottler, Jeffrey A. *The Compleat Therapist*. San Francisco: Jossey-Bass, 1991. p. 10.
27 Dawes, Robyn M. *House of Cards: Psychology and Psychotherapy Built on Myth*. New York: Macmillan, 1994. p. 30.
28 Lambert, M. J. 'Some implications of psychotherapy outcome research for eclectic psychotherapy.' *International Journal of Eclectic Psychotherapy*, 5(1), 1986. pp. 16–44.
29 White, G. D., and Pollard, J. 'Assessing therapeutic competence from therapy session attendance.' *Professional Psychology*, 13, 1982. pp. 628–33.
30 Eysenck, Hans J. 'A mish-mash of theories.' *International Journal of Psychiatry*, 9, 1970, pp. 140–46 (p. 145).
31 Orlinsky, D. E., and Howard, K. I. 'Process outcome in psychotherapy.' In S. L. Garfield and A. E. Bergin (eds.) *Handbook of Psychotherapy and Behaviour Change*. (3rd edn) New York: John Wiley, 1986. For example, Barendregt, J. T. 'A psychological investigation of the effects of psychoanalysis and psychotherapy.' In *Research in Psychodiagnostics*. Paris: Mouton, 1961.

32 For example, Lorr, M., and McNair, D. M. 'Frequency of treatment and change in psychotherapy.' *Journal of Abnormal and Social Psychology*, 64, 1962. pp. 281–92.

33 Task Force for the Promotion and Dissemination of Psychological Procedures, American Psychological Association – Division 12. *The Clinical Psychologist*, May 1995.

34 Criteria: 'A treatment must be supported by research demonstrating efficacy either by showing it is superior to a pill, psychological placebo or another treatment, or showing that the treatment is equivalent to an already established treatment.' *APA Monitor*, March 1995. p. 4.

35 Chambless, Dianne L., et al. 'Update on empirically validated therapies, II.' *Clinical Psychologist*, 51(1), 1998. pp. 3–16.

36 Woody, Sheila R., and Sanderson, William C. 'Manuals for empirically supported treatments: 1998 Update.' Published by APA Division 12.

37 Strupp, Hans, and Hadley, Suzanne. 'Specific versus nonspecific factors in psychotherapy.' *Archives of General Psychiatry*, 36, 1979. pp. 1125–1136.

38 Stein, D. M. and Lambert, M. J. 'On the relationship between therapist experience and psychotherapy outcome.' *Clinical Psychology Review*, 4, 1984. pp. 127–42.

39 See Garb, H. N. 'Clinical judgement, clinical training, and professional experience.' *Psychological Bulletin*, 105, 1989. pp. 387–96.

40 *Report of the Task Force on the Evaluation of Education, Training and Service in Psychology*. Washington, DC: American Psychological Association, 1982. (Italics added.)

41 Smith, M. L. and Glass, G. V. 'Meta-analysis of psychotherapy outcome studies.' *American Psychologist*, 32, 1977. pp. 752–60.

42 Lieberman, M. A., Yalom, I. D., and Miles, M. B. *Encounter Groups: First Facts*. New York: Basic Books, 1973.

43 McCord, Joan. 'Consideration of some effects of a counselling program.' In Susan E. Martin, Lee B. Sechrest and Robin Redner (eds.) *New Directions in the Rehabilitation of Criminal Offenders*. Washington, DC: National Academy Press, 1981. pp. 394–405.

44 Sobel, S. B. 'Throwing the baby out with the bathwater.' *American Psychologist*, 33, 1978. pp. 290–91.

45 Ditman, K. S., Crawford, G. C., and Forgy, E. W. 'A controlled experiment on the use of court probation in the management of the alcohol addict.' *American Journal of Psychiatry*, 124, 1967. pp. 160–63.

46 Peele. *Diseasing of America*. p. 57.

47 Spitzer, R. Cited in Sarason. *Psychology Misdirected.* p. 42.
48 Carkhuff, Robert R. *Helping and Human Relations: A Primer for Lay and Professional Helpers.* New York: Holt, Rinehart & Winston, 1969.
49 Berkowitz, Leonard. 'The case for bottling up rage.' *Psychology Today,* July 1978. p. 24.
50 Bergin, A. E. 'The evaluation of therapeutic outcome.' In A. E. Bergin and S. L. Garfield (eds.) *Handbook of Psychotherapy and Behaviour Change.* New York: John Wiley, 1971. p. 263.
51 Hadley, Suzanne W., and Strupp, Hans F. 'Contemporary view of negative effects of psychotherapy.' *Archives of General Psychiatry* 33, November 1976. pp. 1291–1302.
52 Loftus, Elizabeth, Grant, Brian L., Franklin, Gary M., Parr, Loni, and Brown, Rachel. 'Crime victims' compensation and repressed memory.' A letter to the Mental Health Subcommittee, Crime Victims Compensation Program, Department of Labor and Industries, State of Washington. (Revised Version 5-1-96.) The original letter has never been published.
53 Loftus, E. S. 'Repressed memory accusation: Comment on Gudjonsson.' *Journal of Applied Cognitive Psychology,* 11, 1997. pp. 25–30.
54 Lief, H. I., and Fetkewicz, J. 'Retractors of false memories: the evolution of pseudo-memories.' *Journal of Psychiatry and Law,* 23, 1995, 411–36. p. 432.
55 Robinson, Kathryn. 'The end of therapy.' *Seattle Weekly,* 13 November 1996. See also Susan Sarnoff, *Sanctified Snake Oil.* (In press.)
56 For example, Mahrer, Alvin R. 'Some known effects of psychotherapy and reinterpretation.' *Psychotherapy: Research, Theory and Practice,* 7(3), 1970. pp. 186–91.
57 Kottler. *The Compleat Therapist.* p. 18.
58 A USC professor of psychiatry, Dr Mendel, demonstrated this gullibility in an interesting study with his own patients. He created a group of incorrect, horoscope-like interpretations and then offered them to his patients. Twenty out of the twenty-four were accepted by the patients, who also reported a drop in anxiety as a result. ('The phenomenon of interpretation.' *American Journal of Psychoanalysis,* 24(2), 1964. pp. 184–90.)
59 Strupp, Hans H. 'Needed: A reformulation of the psychotherapeutic influence.' *International Journal of Psychiatry,* 10, 1972. pp. 114–20.
60 Kottler. *The Compleat Therapist.* p. 88.
61 Ibid. pp. 75–76.
62 Guy, J. D. *The Personal Life of the Psychotherapist.* New York: John Wiley, 1987. p. 294.
63 Dawes. *House of Cards.* p. 4.

64 Follette, W. T., and Cummings, N. A. 'Psychiatric services and medical utilization in a prepaid health plan setting.' *Medical Care*, 5, 1967. pp. 25–35.
65 VandenBos, Gary R. (ed.) *Psychotherapy: Practice, Research, Policy*. London: Sage Publications. 1980. p. 18.
66 Schlesinger, Herbert J., Mumford, Emily, and Glass, Gene V. 'Mental health services and medical utilization.' In VandenBos. *Psychotherapy*. p. 89.
67 Ibid. pp. 88–89.
68 Ibid. p. 90.
69 Borus, Jonathan F., Olendzki, Margaret C., Kessler, Larry, Burns, Barbara J., Brandt, Ursula C., Broverman, Carol A., and Henderson, Paul R. 'The "Offset Effect" of mental health treatment on ambulatory medical care utilization and charges.' *Archives of General Psychiatry*, 42, 1985. p. 573.
70 Fraser, J. Scott. 'All that glitters is not always gold: Medical offset effects and managed behavioral health care.' *Professional Psychology: Research and Practice*, 27(4), 1996. pp. 335–44.
71 Glover, Edward. *The Techniques of Psycho-Analysis*. New York: International University Press, 1958.
72 Meehl, P. E. 'Psychology: Does our heterogenous subject matter have any unity?' *Minnesota Psychologist*, Summer 1986. p. 4.
73 Kayla Weiner, PhD, Internet posting, November 1995.
74 Alan H. Roberts recalls 'a special meeting [of the Biofeeedback Research Society] devoted to studies ostensibly showing that males could be taught (through biofeedback techniques) to raise the temperature of their testicles high enough to kill sperm and that this process could be used as a form of birth control'. In Roberts, A. H. 'Biofeedback: Research, training, and clinical roles.' *American Psychologist*, 40, 1985. pp. 938–41, p. 939.
75 Mack, John E. *Abduction: Human Encounters with Aliens*. New York: Charles Scribner's Sons, 1994. pp. 2–3.
76 Mack. *Abduction*. p. 13.
77 Mack, John E. 'Mental health professionals and the Roper Poll.' In B. Hopkins, D. M. Jacobs and R. Westrum, *The UFO Abduction Syndrome: A Report on Unusual Experiences Associated with UFO Abductions, The Roper Organization's Survey of 5,947 Adult Americans*. Las Vegas: Bigelow Holding Co., 1992. p. 15.
78 Ibid. pp. 15–16.
79 Mack, *Abduction*. Preface.
80 CNBC Real Personal, 27 April 1992. Cited by Dawes. *House of Cards*. p. 8.
81 Reiser, Martin. 'Hypnosis as an aid in a homicide investigation.' *American Journal of Clinical Hypnosis*, 17(2), October 1974. p. 85.

82 Sears, R. R. 'Survey of objective studies of psychoanalytic concepts.' Social Science Research Council, New York, Bulletin 51, 1943.
83 Wolfe, Peter H. 'Psychoanalytic research and infantile sexuality.' *International Journal of Psychiatry*, 4(1), July 1967. pp. 61–64.
84 Bruck, Maggie, Ceci, Stephen, and Francouer, Emmett. 'Anatomically detailed dolls do not facilitate Preschoolers' reports of touching: The abstract paper' presented at the 1994 Annual Meeting of the Canadian Pediatric Society, St Johns, Newfoundland.
85 Sears, R. R. 1943.
86 Bass, E., and Davis, L. *The Courage to Heal.* New York: Harper & Row, 1988. p. 22.
87 Cited in Rudy, D. *Becoming Alcoholic: Alcoholics Anonymous and the Reality of Alcoholism*. Carbondale, IL: Southern Illinois University Press, 1986.
88 'Mental health: Does therapy help?' *Consumer Reports*, November 1995. pp. 734–39.
89 Seligman, Martin E. P. 'The effectiveness of psychotherapy: The *Consumer Reports* study.' *American Psychologist*, 50(12), 1995. pp. 965–74.
90 'How is your doctor treating you?' *Consumer Reports*, February 1995. pp. 81–88.
91 Dawes. *House of Cards*. p. 44.
92 Bickman, Leonard. 'A continuum of care: More is not always better.' *American Psychologist*, 51(7), 1996, pp. 689–701. See also Bickman, L., Guthrie, P. R., Foster, E. M., Lambert, E. W., Summerfelt, W. T., Breda, C. S., and Heflinger, C. A. *Evaluating Managed Mental Health Services: The Fort Bragg Experiment*. New York: Plenum, 1995.
93 DeLeon, Patrick H., and Williams, Janice G. 'Evaluation research and public policy formation: Are psychologists collectively willing to accept unpopular findings?' *American Psychologist*, 52(5), 1997. p. 551.
94 Bickman, L., Noser, K., and Summerfelt, W. T. 'Long-term effects of a system of care on children and adolescents.' *Journal of Behavioral Health Services Research*, 1999. And Bickman, L., Summerfelt, W. T., Firth, J., and Douglas, S. 'The Stark County Evaluation Project: Baseline results of a randomized experiment.' In D. Northrup and C. Nixon (ed.), *Evaluating Mental Health Services: How Do Programs for Children 'Work' in the Real World?* (pp. 231–59). Newbury Park, CA: Sage Publications, 1997.
95 Bickman et al. 1997. pp. 1543–48.
96 Hoagwood, Kimberly. 'Interpreting nullity: The Fort Bragg Experiment – A comparative success or failure?' *American Psychologist*, 52(5), 1997. p. 548.

97 Bickman, L., Noser, K., and Summerfelt, W. T. 'Long-term effects of a system of care on children and adolescents.' *Journal of Behavioral Health Services Research* (in press). Bickman, L., Summerfelt, W. T., and Noser, K. 'Comparative outcomes of emotionally disturbed children and adolescents in a system of services and usual care.' *Psychiatric Services*, 48(12), 1997, 1543–48.
98 Weisz, Bhar. 'The effectiveness of traditional child psychotherapy.' Unpublished report of the Center for Mental Health Policy, Vanderbilt University, 1997. See also Weisz, J. R., Han, S. S., and Valeri, S. M. 'More of what? Issues raised by the Fort Bragg study.' *American Psychologist*, 52(5), 1997, 541–45; Weisz, J. R., Weiss, B., and Donenberg, G. R. 'The lab versus the clinics: Effects of child and adolescent psychotherapy.' *American Psychologist*, 47, 1992, 1578–85.
99 Personal communication; see also Salzer, M. S., Bickman, L., and Lambert, E. W. 'Dose-effect relationship in children's psychotherapy services.' *Journal of Consulting and Clinical Psychology* (in press).
100 Feldman, Saul. 'The Fort Bragg Demonstration and Evaluation.' *American Psychologist*, 52(5), 1997. p. 560.
101 Hoagwood. 'Interpreting nullity.' p. 548.
102 O. Hobart Mowrer, PhD, American Psychological Association president. *Crisis in Psychiatry and Religion*. New York: Van Nostrand, 1961.
103 M. B. Parloff, 'Can psychotherapy research guide the policy maker?' *American Psychologist*, 34, 1979. pp. 296–306.
104 Dawes. *House of Cards*. p. 58.
105 Sechrest, L., and Walsh, M. 'Dogma or data: Bragging rights.' *American Psychologist*, 52(5), 1997. p. 536.
106 Seligman, M. *What You Can Change and What You Can't*. New York: Knopf, 1994. p. 8.
107 Farley, Frank. 'From the Heart.' *American Psychologist*, 51(8), 1996. p. 774.

Chapter 4

1 *The Family Therapy Networker*, March/April 1995.
2 President's Column, *APA Monitor*, June 1995. p. 2.
3 Frank. *Persuasion and Healing*. p. 8.
4 Robiner, William N. 'How many psychologists are needed? A call for a national psychology human resource agenda.' *Professional Psychology: Research and Practice*. 22(6), 1991. pp. 427–40.
5 Rome, H. P. 'Psychiatry and Foreign Affairs.' *American Journal of Psychiatry*,

125, 1968, p. 729; and '"The psychiatrist," the American Psychiatric Association, and social issues.' *American Journal of Psychiatry*, 128, 1971, p. 686.
6 Torrey, E. Fuller. *Freudian Fraud: The Malignant Effect of Freud's Theory on American Thought and Culture.* New York: HarperCollins, 1993. p. 129.
7 Smail. *Taking Care.* p. 40.
8 Zilbergeld. *The Shrinking of America.* p. 91.
9 Albee, G. W. 'A competency model must replace the defect model.' In Bond, L. A. and Rosen, J. C. *Competence and Coping During Adulthood.* Thousand Oaks, CA: Sage Publ., 1980. p. 95.
10 Farley, Frank. 'Thrills.' The President's column in the *APA Monitor*, February 1994. p. 3.
11 Stanley Shapiro, director of the Parenting Education Centre in Ontario, quoted in 'Spanking: The discipline dilemma.' *Homemaker's Magazine*, October 1995. p. 50.
12 'Son suing his parents opens a Pandora's box.' *Washington Post*, 1 October 1979, B1.
13 Gross. *The Psychological Society.* p. 267.
14 Westman, Jack C. *Licensing Parents: Can We Prevent Child Abuse and Neglect.* New York: Insight Books, Plenum Press, 1994.
15 Fenster, C. A., et al. 'Careers in forensic psychology.' In Woods, P. J., *Career Opportunities for Psychologists.* Washington: APA, 1976, pp. 124–25.
16 Scott Sleek. 'A varied practice is the key to security.' *APA Monitor*, March 1995. p. 28.
17 Frank Cavaliere. 'Psychology-and-law field well-positioned for growth.' *APA Monitor*, August 1995. p. 43.
18 *Ferguson v. Hubbell*, 97, NY, pp. 507 and 514 (1884). Cited in Huber, *Galileo's Revenge.* p. 13.
19 Ibid. p. 2.
20 Ibid. p. 3.
21 Hagen, Margaret A. *Whores of the Court: The Fraud of Psychiatric Testimony and the Rape of American Justice.* New York: Regan Books, HarperCollins, 1997. p. 301.
22 Hole, Christina. *Witchcraft in England.* New York: Collier Books, 1966. pp. 75, 89.
23 Mackay, C. *Extraordinary Popular Delusions and the Madness of the Crowds* (1841). New York: Noonday Press, 1962. p. 481.
24 See Lindsay, D. S., Johnson, M. K., and Kwon, P. 'Developmental changes in memory source monitoring.' *Journal of Experimental Child Psychology*, 52, 1991, pp. 297–318; White, S., and Quinn, K. M. 'Investigatory independence

in child sexual abuse evaluations: Conceptual considerations ' *Bulletin of the American Academy of Psychiatry and the Law*, 16(3), 1988, pp. 269–78; Campbell, Terence W. 'False allegations of sexual abuse and the persuasiveness of play therapy.' In press; and Gabriel, Ronald M. 'Anatomically correct dolls in the diagnosis of sexual abuse of children.' *Journal of the Melanie Klein Society*. 3(2), 1985. pp. 40–51.

25 Margolin, K. N. 'How shall facilitated communication be judged? Facilitated communication and the legal system.' In H. C. Shane (ed.) *Facilitated Communication: The Clinical and Social Phenomenon*. San Diego, CA: Singular Press, 1994. pp. 227–58.

26 Jacobson, John W., Mulick, James A., and Schwartz, Allen A. 'A History of facilitated communication: Science, pseudoscience, and antiscience working group on facilitated communication.' *American Psychologist*, 50(9), 1995. pp. 750–65.

27 Gardner, Richard A. 'The "Validators" and other examiners.' *Issues in Child Abuse Accusations*. 3(1), 1991. pp. 38–39.

28 A letter from Carol L. Hopkins, deputy foreman of the 1991–92 San Diego County Grand Jury studying the California juvenile dependency system, to the Honourable Henry J. Hyde, chairman of the House Judiciary Committee, Washington, DC. See also Nathan, Debbie, and Snedeker, Michael J. *Satan's Silence: Ritual Abuse and the Making of a Modern American Witchhunt*. New York: HarperCollins, 1995.

29 Lasch, Christopher. *Haven in a Heartless World: The Family Besieged*. New York: Basic Books, 1997. p. 136.

30 Zimbardo, Philip G., and Radl, Shirley. *The Shy Child: A Parent's Guide to Overcoming and Preventing Shyness from Infancy to Adulthood*. New York: McGraw-Hill Books, 1981. pp. 26–27.

31 Ruesch, Jurgen, and Bateson, Gregory. *Communication: The Social Matrix of Psychiatry*. New York: Norton, 1951. p. 71.

32 Marone. *Women and Risk*. p. 7.

33 APA past president Ronald Fox, quoted in 'Fox identifies top threats to professional psychology,' by Sara Martin in the *APA Monitor*, March 1995. p. 44.

34 Schaef, *Beyond Therapy, Beyond Science*. p. 94.

35 Pittman, Frank, III. 'A buyer's guide to psychotherapy.' *Psychology Today*, Jan/Feb 1994. pp. 52–53.

36 Rosenberg, Jerry M. *The Dictionary of Marketing and Advertising*. New York: John Wiley, 1995. p. 122.

37 Marone. *Women and Risk*. p. xiii.

38 Barnett-Queen, Timothy, and Bergmann, Lawrence H. 'Response to traumatic event crucial in preventing lasting consequences.' *Occupational Health and Safety*, July 1990. pp. 53–55.
39 Elgin, Suzette Haden. *You Can't Say That to Me!: Stopping the Pain of Verbal Abuse – An 8-Step Program*. New York: John Wiley, 1995. pp. 2–3.
40 Harris, Scott, and Reynolds, Edward. *When Growing Up Hurts Too Much*. New York: Lexington Books (Macmillan), 1990. p. 70.
41 Marone. *Women and Risk*. p. xiv.
42 'Beyond Perfect Health.' Cited by Zilbergeld, *The Shrinking of America*. p. 92.
43 Polster, Irving and Miriam, *Gestalt Therapy Integrated*. 1973. p. 91.
44 Szasz. *The Myth of Psychotherapy*. p. 194.
45 Schaef, Anne W. *When Society Becomes an Addict*. San Francisco: Harper and Row, 1987. p. 18.
46 Jeffers, Susan. *Dare to Connect*. New York: Ballantine, 1992.
47 Beattie, Melody. *Codependent No More*. New York: Harper and Row, 1989. p. 26.
48 Jeffers. *Dare to Connect*. p. 46.
49 Schaef, Anne W. *Co-Dependence: Misunderstood, Mistreated*. San Francisco: Harper and Row, 1986. p. 67.
50 Attributed to Peter Vegso, Health Communications, Inc. Cited by Kaminer, Wendy. *I'm Dysfunctional, You're Dysfunctional*. New York: Vintage Books, 1993. p. 12.
51 Bradshaw. *Bradshaw On*. Deerfield Beach, FL: Health Communications, 1996. p. 180.
52 Ricketson, Susan Coley. *The Dilemma of Love: Healing Co-dependent Relationships at Different Stages of Life*. Deerfield Beach, Fl: Health Communications, 1989. p. 13.
53 Kaminer. *I'm Dysfunctional, You're Dysfunctional*. p. 10.
54 Branden, N. 'In defense of self.' *Association of Humanistic Psychology Perspectives*, 8–9, 1984. p. 12.
55 Harris and Edward. *When Growing Up Hurts Too Much*. p. 70.
56 Taylor, S. *Positive Illusions: Creative Self-Deception and the Healthy Mind*. New York: Basic Books, 1989. p. 227.
57 For a more thorough review of the task-force report, *The Social Importance of Self-Esteem* (1989), see Dawes. *House of Cards*. pp. 236–51.
58 Mecca, A. M., Smelser, N. J., and Vasconcellos, J. *The Social Importance of Self-Esteem*. Berkeley: University of California Press, 1989. p. 15.
59 Bhatti, B., Derezotes, D., Kim, S. O. and Specht, H. 'The association

between child maltreatment and self-esteem.' In Mecca et al. *The Social Importance of Self-Esteem*. pp. 24–71.
60 Woititz, J. G. 'A study of self-esteem in children of alcoholics.' PhD dissertation, Rutgers University, 1976. pp. 53–55.
61 'BPA Retreat focuses on the changing environment.' *APA Monitor*, February 1997.
62 The working definition of Emerge, a Boston counselling programme for men who batter. Cited in Jones, Ann. *Next Time, She'll Be Dead: Battering and How to Stop It*. Boston: Beacon Press, 1994.
63 For instance, 1998 homicide rates in the United States were the lowest they have been since 1967, with cities like New York showing a 47 per cent decrease in the past eight years.
64 *Violence and Youth: Psychology's Response. Volume I: Summary Report of the American Psychological Association Commission on Violence and Youth*. Washington, DC: American Psychological Association, 1993. p. 14.
65 James Q. Wilson and Richard J. Herrnstein in their book *Crime and Human Nature*; Robert ten Bensel, director, Maternal and Child Health, the University of Minnesota, attributed to Richard Gelles. Both cited by the Honourable Anne C. Cools, Senator, on 30 March 1995, during the first session of the 35th Canadian Parliament, Vol. 135. p. 1496.
66 William Coleman, a Vancouver psychologist, quoted when speaking about a sex offender released into the community after serving his prison sentence. *Times Colonist*, 16 August 1995.
67 Cited in the section on domestic violence in *No Safe Haven, the Report of the APA Task Force on Male Violence Against Women*. Washington, DC: American Psychological Association, 1994.
68 Such a programme was ordered by the Nevada Supreme Court, citing 'near-epidemic proportions of violence against women nationally'. All courts were closed for a day (18 or 19 October 1993) and judges were ordered to attend a seminar on domestic violence.
69 Becker, Judith, cited in the *APA Monitor*, 25(1), January 1994. p. 1.
70 Sleet, Scott. 'Prevention is worth pounds of penalties.' *APA Monitor*, 25 (1), January 1994. p. 1.
71 Nelson, J. A. 'The impact of incest: Factors in self-evaluation.' In L. L. Constantine and F. M. Martinson (ed.) *Children and Sex: New Findings, New Perspectives*. Boston: Little, Brown, 1981. pp. 163–74.
72 Burgess, A. W., and Hartman, C. R. 'Sex rings, pornography, and prostitution.' In S. Ludwig and A. E. Kornberg (ed.) *Child Abuse: A Medical Reference*. New York: Churchill Livingstone, 1992. p. 298.

73 Levitt, E. E., and Pinnell, C. M. 'Some additional light on the childhood sexual abuse–psychopathology axis.' *International Journal of Clinical and Experimental Hypnosis*, 43(2), April 1995. p. 148.
74 Ibid. pp. 149–50.
75 Elgin, Suzette Hagen. *You Can't Say That to Me!* p. 109.
76 Cited in Richard Lacayo's article 'Assault by paragraph.' *Time*, 17 January 1994. p. 37.
77 Fatalities for 1986 were 1,014 and for 1993 they were 1,216, according to the National Committee to Prevent Child Abuse.
78 Blyskal, Jeff. 'Head Hunt: How to find the right psychotherapist – for the right price.' *New York*, 11 January 1993. p. 29.
79 Marilyn Murray is cited in Beigel, Joan Kaye, and Earle, Ralph H. *Successful Private Practice in the 1990s: A New Guide for the Mental Health Professional.* New York: Brunner/Mazel, 1990. p. 83.
80 Jones. *Next Time, She'll Be Dead.* p. 1.
81 Schaef. *Beyond Therapy, Beyond Science.* p. 91.
82 Lisa Rabasca. 'Finding the right niche in the new market.' *APA Monitor*, February 1999. p. 1.
83 Grinker, Roy R., and Spiegel, John P. *Men Under Stress.* New York: McGraw-Hill, 1945.
84 For example, Holmes, T. H., and Rahe, R. H. 'The Social Readjustment Rating Scale.' *Journal of Psychosomatic Research*, 11, 1967, pp. 213–18. For more, consult Miller, T. W. (ed.) *Stressful Life Events.* Madison, Conn: International Universities Press, 1989.
85 For example, Winter, Richard E. (ed.) *Coping with Executive Stress.* New York: McGraw-Hill, 1983.
86 For example, Meichenbaum, Donald. *Coping with Stress.* Toronto: John Wiley, 1983.
87 *Prisoner of Childhood* was the original title of Alice Miller's first book, translated by Ruth Ward. New York: Basic Books, 1981. Reissued as *The Drama of the Gifted Child.* New York: Basic Books, 1982.
88 Zilbergeld illustrates the media's bias in describing the experience of Curtiss Anderson, once an editor of *Ladies' Home Journal*:

> The Journal had done a series of articles on women who had dieted, lost lots of weight, and gone on to fulfil their dreams: marriage, children, and homes in the suburbs. Anderson decided to do a follow-up, which was approved by chief editor Beatrice Gould, who thought it would show the women 'living happily ever after.' But this is not what was found. According

to Anderson, 'Ninety-nine percent had blown right back up to their old weights. They'd lost their husbands, been divorced, and they were angry again.' Anderson thought he had an important story on the meaninglessness of the *Journal*'s stories and diets. But it was never published. Mrs Gould was appalled. She didn't want to hear about it. 'I don't believe it,' she said.

Zilbergeld, B. *The Shrinking of America*. p. 106.
89 Ries, A., and Trout, J. *The 22 Immutable Laws of Marketing*. New York: HarperBusiness, 1993. p. 10.
90 Quoted from Internet communications from Charles Figley, founding chair of the Green Cross, July 1995.
91 'Counselling "does more harm than good"' by David Fletcher, health correspondent, *Daily Telegraph* (London), 27 September 1997.
92 Personal communication, November 1997.
93 'Coffee-cup therapy' is a term that psychologists use to describe their work as they are 'simply talking to survivors as they go about their business'. It is also referred to as 'stealth psychology' because they do not identify themselves as mental-health professionals. (See Rebecca Clay. 'Psychologists help flood victims to cope.' *APA Monitor*, July 1997. p. 23.)
94 'Disaster victims need more long-term care, report says.' *APA Monitor*, October 1997. p. 18.
95 Salzer, Mark S., and Bickman, Leonard. 'The short- and long-term psychological impact of disasters: Implications for mental health interventions and policy.' In Gist, R. M. and Lubin, B. (eds.) *Response to Disaster: Psychosocial, Ecological and Community Approaches*. Philadelphia: Taylor & Francis (in press).
96 Poak, Paul R., Egan, Donald, Vadenbergh, Richard, and Williams, W. Vail. 'Prevention in mental health: A controlled study.' *American Journal of Psychiatry*, 132(2), 1975. pp. 146–49.
97 Mitchell, J. T. 'Recovery from rescue.' *Response: The Magazine of Rescue and Emergency Management*, Fall 1982, pp. 7–10; and Mitchell, J. T., and Resnick, H. *Emergency Response to Crisis*. Bowie, Maryland: Robert J. Brady, 1981.
98 Tvedten, J. 'Critical incident stress debriefing: What is it and how can you use it?' *Commish*, 4(2), 1994. p. 7.
99 See Gist and Lubin. *Response to Disaster*; Gist, R., and Woodall, S. J. 'Social science versus social movements: The origins and natural history of debriefing.' *Australasian Journal of Disaster and Trauma Studies*, 1, 1998.
100 Information is derived from an article by Elizabeth Gleick, 'Tower of psychobabble.' *Time*, 16 June 1997. pp. 69–73.
101 Walker, I., and Broderick, P. 'The psychology of assisted reproduction,

or psychology assisting its reproduction?' Submitted to the *Australian Psychologist* 1997; available from Dr Iain Walker, Psychology Dept., Murdoch University, Murdoch, WA, 6150, Australia.

102 Humphrey, M., Humphrey, H., and Ainsworth, I. 'Screening couples for parenthood by donor insemination.' *Social Sciences and Medicine*, 32, 1991. pp. 273–78.

103 Ley, P. 'Reproductive technology – What can we learn from the adoption experience?' In Swain, P., and Swain, S. (ed.) *To Search for Self*, Sydney: Federation Press, 1992. pp. 100–10; Turner, C. 'A call for openness in donor insemination.' *Politics and the Life Sciences*, 12, 1993. pp. 197–99.

104 Western Australia Human Reproductive Technology Council. *Questions and Answers about the Donation of Human Reproductive Material*. Perth: Health Department of Western Australia, 1995.

105 Daniels, K. R., and Taylor, K. 'Secrecy and openness in donor insemination.' *Politics and the Life Sciences*, 12, 1993. p. 158.

106 Snowden, R., and Mitchell, G. D. *The Artificial Family: A Consideration of Artificial Insemination by Donor*. London: Allen & Unwin, 1981.

107 Walker and Broderick. 'The psychology of assisted reproductions.' p. 16.

108 Daniels, K., and Stjerna, I. 'Infertility: The social work contribution.' *Socionomen*, 6, 1993. pp. 41–46.

109 Schwarzchild, Michael. 'Why I changed my mind on prescribing.' *APA Monitor*, February 1997. p. 19.

110 'Helping to secure Rx privileges.' *APA Monitor*, September 1996.

111 DeLeon, Patrick H., and Wiggins, Jack G. Jr. 'Prescription privileges for psychologists.' *American Psychologist*, 51(3), 1996. pp. 225, 228.

112 DeNelsky, G. Y. 'The case against prescription privileges for psychologists.' *American Psychologist*, 51(3), 1996. p. 207.

113 'Prozac prophet.' The cover story of *Maclean's*, 23 May 1994. p. 41.

114 Levine, Judith. 'A question of abuse.' *Mother Jones*, July–August 1996.

115 Cited by Levine in 'A question of abuse'.

116 Levine, Judith. *In Search of Innocence: America's Battle Over Children's Sexuality*. New York: Houghton-Mifflin, 1998.

117 Again cited by Levine in 'A question of abuse'.

118 A publication of the Practice Directorate of the American Psychological Association describing the 'APA Disaster Response Network', p. 1. (Italics added.)

119 A publication of the Practice Directorate of the APA on 'Diversifying Your Sources of Practice Income'. p. 1.

120 72.8 per cent provide pro bono mental-health services, and 65.7 per cent provide other services pro bono. From the *Profile of All Members: 1993*. Office of Demographic, Employment, and Educational Research, APA Education Directorate.

121 Suicide: 'It is important for all survivors to understand what they are going through, to recognize the symptoms that are part of grieving after suicide, part of Posttraumatic Stress Disorder.' From Lukas, C., and Seiden, H. M., *Silent Grief: Living in the Wake of Suicide*. New York: Macmillan, 1987, p. 42; Pets: Quackenbush, Jamie. *When Your Pet Dies: How to Cope With Your Feelings*. New York: Simon and Schuster, 1985; Death: Akner, Lois F. *How to Survive the Loss of a Parent*. New York: William Morrow, 1993; Veterans: Beal, Lynne A. 'Post-traumatic stress disorder in prisoners of war and combat veterans of the Dieppe raid: A 50-year follow-up.' *Canadian Journal of Psychiatry*, 40, 1995, pp. 177–84; and Gender: A woman claimed discrimination by the Anglican Church as the reason she was never ordained a priest. In court, a psychologist stated that she was 'suffering from post-traumatic stress disorder, because of her treatment by the church, which left her feeling "shunned, humiliated and victimized"'. *Victoria Times Colonist*, 25 February 1995. pp. 1, 6.

122 Love: 'Addiction has as much to do with love as it does with drugs. Many of us are addicts, only we don't know it.' Peele, Stanton, and Brodsky, Archie. *Love and Addiction*. New York: Signet, 1975. p. 1; Sex: Robinson, Barbara L., and Robinson, Rick L. *If My Dad's a Sexaholic, What Does that Make Me?* Minneapolis, Minn.: CompCare, 1992; 'Urgency': Tassi, Nina. *Urgency Addiction: How to Slow Down without Sacrificing Success*. New York: Signet, 1991; Religion: 'No addiction is more toxically shaming and soul-murdering than the religious abuse that flows from the actions of religious addicts.' John Bradshaw in the Foreword to Father Leo Booth's book *When God Becomes a Drug: Breaking the Chains of Religious Addiction and Abuse – Attaining Healthy Spirituality*. Los Angeles: Jeremy P. Tarcher, 1992; Shopping: Damon, Janet E. *Shopaholics: An 8-Week Program to Control Compulsive Shopping*. New York: Avon Books, 1988; On-Line: O'Neill, Molly. 'The lure and addiction of life on line.' *New York Times*, 8 March 1995; Food: Karen Russell, a recovered overeater who claims to have lost 300 pounds, presents one-and-a-half-day seminars entitled 'Reclaiming Your Life' to professionals and individuals concerned with emotional eating; and Prostitution: 'Prostitution is not an option for women but an addiction that requires long-range support and encouragement for cure.' Samuel S. Janus, PhD, 'Prostitution called an addiction requiring long-term treatment.' *Clinical Psychiatry News*, 5 June 1977. p. 12.

123 Siegel, Micki. 'The power of pets.' *Good Housekeeping*, November 1995. p. 26.

124 'Calming llamas.' *The Therapist*, 4(3), 1997. p. 7.
125 Figley, Charles. 'Compassion fatigue.' Edwards, Randall, '"Compassion fatigue": when listening hurts.' *APA Monitor*, September 1995. p. 34.
126 'Certification in Accelerated Recovery for Compassion Fatigue.' The Traumatology Institute. (www.cpd.fsu.edu/pet/trauma-1b.htm)
127 Holdings, Reynold. 'Sick and twisted system.' *San Francisco Chronicle*, 18 May 1997.
128 'You've got mail, and it's driving you crazy.' *National Post*, 19 January 1999, A1.
129 Miami, Florida. 6 January. PRNewswire.
130 'Cognitive Therapy: A Multimedia Learning Program' at mindstreet.com.
131 Dr Razzaque is fully registered with the General Medical Council of the UK and currently an inceptor of the Royal College of Psychiatry of the UK. His services were announced with the launch of CyberAnalysis.com.
132 Shalit, Ruth. 'Dysfunction Junction.' *New Republic*, 14 April 1997.
133 Kottler, J. *On Being a Therapist*. p. 108.
134 Janet, Pierre. *Psychological Healing: A Historical and Clinical Study*. Vol. II, translated by Eden and Cedar Paul, New York: Macmillan, 1925. p. 338.
135 'Thus, does deception become the cornerstone of modern medical psychotherapeutics.' Szasz, *The Myth of Psychotherapy*. p. 195.
136 Kottler, J. *On Being a Therapist*. p. 108.
137 The journalist Bruce Grearson, personal communication; this comment was reportedly made by Dr Lawrence Pazder, co-author of *Michelle Remembers*.
138 See Gardner, Richard A. 'The "Validators" and other examiners.' *Issues in Child Abuse Accusations*, 3(1), 1991. pp. 38–53.
139 Transcribed from the tape recording of the presentation of Alan Scheflin, JD, LLM, at the Frontiers of Hypnosis conference: the Fourth National Assembly of the Federation of Canadian Societies of Clinical Hypnosis held at Banff, Canada, 4–9 May 1995.
140 Scheflin, Alan. 'Hypnosis 1994 and beyond.' *Hypnos*, 21(4), 1994. p. 202.
141 Sharaf, Myron R., and Levinson, Daniel. 'The quest for omnipotence in professional training.' *International Journal of Psychiatry*, 4(5), 1967. pp. 426–42. Cited in Gross, p. 45.
142 Arons, Gina, and Siegel, Ronald D. 'Unexpected encounters: The Wizard of OZ exposed.' In Sussman, Michael B. (ed.) *A Perilous Calling: The Hazards of Psychotherapy Practice*. New York: Wiley Interscience, 1995. p. 125.
143 Ibid. p. 131.
144 Smail. *Taking Care*. p. 128.
145 Kottler. *On Being a Therapist*. p. 65.

Chapter 5

1 Wolfe, Thomas. 'The "Me" decade.' *New York*, 23 August 1976, p. 30.

2 Strupp, Hans H. 'Needed: A reformulation of the psychotherapeutic influence.' *International Journal of Psychiatry*, 26, March 1972, pp.270–78.

3 Slaby. *Aftershock*. pp. 4–5.

4 Ibid. p. 217 (the last page of the book).

5 Frank. *Persuasion and Healing*. p. 216.

6 Calestro, Kenneth M. 'Psychotherapy, faith healing and suggestion.' *International Journal of Psychiatry*, 10, 1972, pp. 83–113. See also Whitman, Roy M. 'Which dreams does the patient tell?' *Archives of General Psychiatry*, 8, 1963. pp. 277–82.

7 Welkowitx, J., Cohen, J., and Ortmeyer, D. 'Value system similarity: Investigation of patient–therapist dyads.' *Journal of Consulting Psychology*, 31, 1967. pp. 48–55.

8 Rosenthal, D. 'Changes in some moral values following psychotherapy.' *Journal of Consulting Psychology*, 19, 1955. pp. 431–36.

9 Lynn, S. J., and Rhue, J. W. 'Fantasy-proneness: Hypnosis, developmental antecedents, and psychopathology.' *American Psychologist*, 43, 1988, pp. 35–44.

10 Maltz, Wendy. *The Sexual Healing Journey: A Guide for Survivors of Sexual Abuse*. San Francisco: HarperCollins, 1992.

11 Zelig, M., and Beidleman, W. 'The investigative use of hypnosis: A word of caution.' *International Journal of Clinical and Experimental Hypnosis*, 29, 1981. pp. 401–12.

12 Bryant, Richard A. 'Fantasy-proneness, reported childhood abuse, and the relevance of reported abuse onset.' *International Journal of Clinical and Experimental Hypnosis*, 43, 1995. pp. 184–93.

13 Borch-Jacobsen, Mikkel. 'Sybil – the making of a disease: An interview with Dr Herbert Spiegel.' *New York Review*, 24, 1997. p. 62.

14 Kardiner, Abram. *My Analysis with Freud*. New York: Norton, 1977. p. 75.

15 Saul Bellow in his Foreword to Allan Bloom's *The Closing of the American Mind*. New York: Touchstone Books (Simon and Schuster), 1987.

16 Bloom. *The Closing of the American Mind*. p. 360.

17 Holmes, T. H., and Rahe, R. H. 'The Social Readjustment Rating Scale.' *Journal of Psychosomatic Research*, 11, 1967. pp. 213–18.

18 For reviews, see Miller, Thomas W. (ed.) *Stressful Life Events*. Madison, Conn.: International Universities Press, Stress and Health Series, Monograph

4, 1989; Stone, G. C., Cohen, F., and Adler, N. E. *Health Psychology – A Handbook.* San Francisco: Jossey-Bass, 1979. pp. 77–111.

19 Friedman, M. and Rosenman, R. H. *Type A Behavior and Your Heart.* New York: Knopf, 1974.

20 Rosenman, R. H., and Chesney, M. A. 'Type A behavior and coronary heart disease.' In C. D. Spielberger, I. G. Sarason, and P. B. Defares (eds.) *Stress and Anxiety*, Vol. 9. Washington, DC: Hemisphere, 1985. pp. 207–29.

21 Pious, Scott. *The Psychology of Judgment and Decision-Making.* New York: McGraw, 1993. pp. 162–67; and Piattelli-Palmarini, Massimo. *Inevitable Illusions: How Mistakes of Reason Rule Our Mind.* New York: John Wiley, 1994. pp. 120–23.

22 Dantzer. *The Psychosomatic Delusion.* p. 153.

23 Matthew, K. A. 'Coronary heart disease and Type A behaviors: Update on an alternative to the Booth-Kewley and Friedman (1987) quantitative review.' *Psychological Bulletin*, 104, 1988. pp. 373–80.

24 Parloff, Morris. Cited in Gross. *The Psychological Society.* p. 30.

25 Kubler-Ross, Elizabeth. *On Death and Dying.* New York: Alfred Knopf, 1981.

26 Wortman and Silver. *Journal of Consulting and Clinical Psychology*, Vol. 57, 1989. pp. 349–57.

27 Pennebaker, James W. *Opening Up: The Healing Power of Confiding in Others.* New York: William Morrow, 1990. p. 97.

28 Stroebe, Margaret and Wolfgang. *Handbook of Bereavement: Theory, Research, and Intervention.* Cambridge: Cambridge University Press, 1993.

29 Nussbaum, Emily. 'Good grief! The case for repression.' *Lingua Franca*, October 1997. pp. 48–51.

30 Quackenbush, Jamie. *When Your Pet Dies: How to Cope with Your Feelings.* New York: Simon & Schuster, 1985. Quotes from the jacket cover.

31 Weatherhead, L. D. *Psychology, Religion and Healing.* New York: Abingdon Press, 1952 (revised edn). pp. 122–28.

32 Bergin, Allen, and Garfield, Sol L. (eds.) *Handbook of Psychotherapy and Behavioral Change: An Empirical Analysis.* New York: John Wiley, 1971 (4th edn 1993). p. 827.

33 Peele. *Diseasing of America.* p. 4.

34 Holden, C. 'The neglected disease in medical education.' *Science*, 229, 1985. pp. 741–42.

35 Conrad, Peter, and Schneider, Joseph W. *Deviance and Medicalization: From Badness to Sickness.* St Louis, Missouri: C. V. Mosby, 1980. p. viii.

36 A publication of Straight Inc. Cited by Peele. *Diseasing of America*, p. 51.
37 Damon, Janet E. *Shopaholics: An 8-Week Program to Control Compulsive Shopping*. New York: Avon Books, 1988. p. 3 and jacket cover.
38 *Star Trek* fans are like drug addicts who suffer withdrawal symptoms if deprived of their favourite television show, a British comedian, Sandy Wolfson, says. 'My research found that about five to ten percent of fans met the psychological criteria of addiction.'
39 The psychologist Marvin Steinberg says: 'Some people may now have an addiction to the stock-market every bit as dangerous as compulsive gambling at casinos or racetracks.' *Canadian Press*, 6 June 1997.
40 Rudy, D. *Becoming Alcoholic: Alcoholics Anonymous and the Reality of Alcoholism*. Carbondale, IL: Southern Illinois University Press, 1986.
41 'United and conquer.' *Newsweek*, 5 February 1990. p. 50.
42 Kaminer. *I'm Dysfunctional, You're Dysfunctional.*
43 M. Freudenheim, 'Business and health: Acknowledging substance abuse.' *New York Times*, 13 December 1988. p. D2.
44 Peele. *Diseasing of America*. p. 52.
45 An unpublished study by the Addiction Research Foundation of Ontario, Toronto, Canada, by the sociologist Sandra Aylward, 1994.
46 Rutter, Peter. *Sex in The Forbidden Zone: When Men in Power – Therapists, Doctors, Clergy, Teachers, and Others – Betray Women's Trust*. New York: Fawcett Crest, 1989. p. 197.
47 'The It's-Not-My-Fault Syndrome.' *US News and World Report*, 18 June 1990. p. 16.
48 Miller, Alice. *Thou Shalt Not Be Aware: Society's Betrayal of the Child*. Trans. by Hildegarde and Hunter Hannum. New York: Farrar, Strauss, Giroux, 1984. pp. 316–17.
49 Miller, Alice. *Banished Knowledge: Facing Childhood Injuries*. Trans. by Leile Vennewitz. New York: Doubleday, 1990. See pp. 181–89.
50 This view is at odds with Freud's personal explanation of the events:

> Under the pressure of the technical procedure which I used at the time, the majority of my patients reproduced from their childhood scenes in which they were sexually seduced by some grown-up person . . . I believed these stories, and consequently supposed that I had discovered the roots of the subsequent neurosis in these experiences of sexual seduction in childhood . . . When, however, I was at last obliged to recognize that these scenes of seduction had never taken place, and that they were only phantasies which my patients had made up or which I myself had perhaps forced upon them,

I was for some time completely at a loss. My confidence alike in my technique and in its results suffered a severe blow . . .

Freud, Sigmund, *An Autobiographical Study*. Trans. by James Strachey. London: Leonard and Virginia Woolf, Institute of Psycho-Analysis, 1936. pp. 60–61.

51 Dolan, Yvonne M. *Resolving Sexual Abuse: Solution-Focused Therapy and Ericksonian Hypnosis for Adult Survivors*. New York: W. W. Norton & Co., 1991. p. 5.

52 Cited in 'Lies of the mind'. *Time*, 29 November 1993. p. 57.

53 Blume, E. Sue. *Secret Survivors: Uncovering Incest and Its Aftereffects in Women*. New York: John Wiley, 1990. p. 78.

54 Friesen, James G. *Uncovering the Mystery of MPD – Its Shocking Origins . . . Its Surprising Cure*. San Bernardino, CA: Here's Life Publishers, 1991.

55 Blume. *Secret Survivors*. p. 81.

56 Williams, M. H. 'The bait-and-switch tactic in psychotherapy.' *Psychotherapy*, 22, 1985. p. 111.

57 Blume. *Secret Survivors*. pp. xviii–xx.

58 Whitfield. *Healing the Child Within*. pp. 3–4.

59 Cited by Smith, Susan E. 'Body memories: And other pseudo-scientific notions of "survivors psychology".' *Issues in Child Abuse Accusations*, 5(4), 1993. pp. 220–34.

60 Cited in 'Lies of the Mind'. *Time*, 29 November 1993. p. 57.

61 Herman. *Trauma and Recovery*. p. 176.

62 Blume. *Secret Survivors*. p. 106.

63 Herman, p. 177; concurring with McCann, L., and Pearlman, L. *Psychological Trauma and the Adult Survivor: Theory, Therapy and Transformation*. New York: Brunner/Mazel, 1990.

64 The terminology of John Bradshaw, Charles Whitfield, Alice Miller, many hypnotists, and Sue Blume, respectively.

65 Bass and Davis. *Courage to Heal*. p. 154.

66 'Devilish Deeds.' ABC News Primetime Live, 7 January 1993. (Transcript 279)

67 Smith. *Survivor Psychology*. p. 19.

68 Described on 'I can't hide my painful secrets anymore'. The Sally Jessy Raphael Show, 22 October 1992. (Transcript 1078)

69 Coleman, Lee. 'Creating "memories" of sexual abuse.' *Issues of Child Abuse Allegations*, 4(4), 1992. pp. 169–76.

70 Herman. *Trauma and Recovery*. p. 158.

71 Stated on ABC News Primetime Live, 7 January 1993.

72 Herman. *Trauma and Recovery*. p. 179.
73 Nisbet, Robert. *History of the Idea of Progress*. New York: Basic Books, 1979. p. 323.
74 Blume. *Secret Survivors*. pp. 78–79.
75 Ibid. p. 130.
76 Bass and Davis. *Courage to Heal*. p. 122.
77 Ibid. p. 124.
78 Herman. *Trauma and Recovery*. p. 178.
79 Bass and Davis. *Courage to Heal*. p. 150.
80 Ibid. p. 318.
81 Herman. *Trauma and Recovery*. p. 210.
82 Bass and Davis quoting Mary R. Williams. *Courage to Heal*. p. 319.
83 Interview, 22 November 1995.
84 Rutter. *Sex in the Forbidden Zone*. p. 28.
85 Dawes. *House of Cards*. p. 58.
86 *American Psychological Association Practitioner Update*, 3(2), June 1995. p. 2.
87 Ralph, Diana. *Work and Madness: The Rise of Community Psychiatry*. Montreal: Black Rose Books, 1983. p. 63.
88 Taylor, F. W. *The Principles of Scientific Management*. New York: W. W. Norton, 1967. p. 125.
89 Peele. *Diseasing of America*. p. 76.
90 Borch-Jacobsen, 1997. p. 64.
91 Edited transcript of remarks by Alan D. Gold, barrister, before the Honourable Senator Anne C. Cools. 10 June 1995, in Toronto, Canada.
92 Stated on ABC Primetime News Live, 7 January 1993. (Transcript 279, p. 3.)
93 Personal communication, November 1995.
94 Kottler. *On Being a Therapist*. p. 17.
95 Kottler. *The Compleat Therapist*. p. 75.

Chapter 6

1 One exception worth reading is: Herman, Ellen. *The Romance of American Psychology: Political Culture in the Age of Experts*. Berkeley, CA: University of California Press, 1995.
2 Schultz, Duane P. *A History of Modern Psychology*. New York: Academic Press, 1969. p. 10.
3 'Social responsibilities of psychologists.' In May, Rollo. *Psychology and the Human Dilemma*. New York: W. W. Norton, 1967.

4 Sarason, Seymour B. *Psychology Misdirected.* New York: Free Press, 1981. p. 154.
5 Galton, Francis. *Hereditary Genius.* London: Macmillan, 1869.
6 The hereditarians' belief that genes are the crucial determinants of human behaviour had been connected to a belief in the inequality of humankind. This included political inequity, a conclusion that Galton himself had clearly expressed. Torrey, E. Fuller. *Freudian Fraud: The malignant effect of Freud's theory on American thought and culture.* New York: HarperCollins, 1993, p. 56.
7 Herrnstein, Richard J., and Murray, Charles. *The Bell Curve: Intelligence and Class Structure in American Life.* New York: Free Press, 1994. p. 5 (Holmes quote: *Buck v. Bell*, 1927).
8 Sarason. *Psychology Misdirected.* p. 74.
9 Herrnstein and Murray wrote: '. . . the use of tests endured and grew because society's largest institutions – schools, military forces, industries, governments – depend significantly on measurable individual differences.' p. 6.
10 Sarason. *Psychology Misdirected.* p. 84.
11 Brown, E. Richard. *Rockefeller Medicine Men: Medicine and Capitalism in America.* Berkeley, CA: University of California Press, 1979. pp. 62–63.
12 Oppenheim, Janet. *'Shattered Nerves'. Doctors, Patients, and Depression in Victorian England.* Oxford: Oxford University Press, 1991.
13 For example, Frederick Nietzsche had written that 'every extension of knowledge arises from making conscious the unconscious.'
14 G. Stanley Hall to Sigmund Freud, 7 October 1909, Clark University Papers. Cited in Turkle, Sherry. *Psychoanalytic Politics: Freud's French Revolution.* New York: Basic Books, 1978. p. 30.
15 Turkle. *Psychoanalytic Politics.* p. 31.
16 Ibid. p. 7.
17 Jacques Lacan, 'The direction of the treatment.' *Ecrits: A Selection*, Trans. by Alan Sheridan. New York: W. W. Norton, 1977. p. 231.
18 Brown. *Rockefeller Medicine Men.* p. 73.
19 Koffka, Kurt. *Principles of Gestalt Psychology.* New York: Harcourt, Brace, Jovanovich, 1935. p. 18.
20 Bingham, W. V. 'Management's concern with research in industrial psychology.' *Harvard Business Review*, 10(1), 1931, p. 52.
21 *The Human Problems of an Industrial Civilization* (1933) and *The Social Problems of an Industrial Civilization* (1945).
22 See Roesthlisberger, F. J. *Management and Morale.* Cambridge, Mass.: Harvard University Press, 1941. p. 16.
23 See Ralph. *Work and Madness.* p. 76; Carey, A. 'The Hawthorne studies:

A radical criticism.' *American Sociological Review*, 1967, 32(3), pp. 403–16; Landsberger, H. A. *Hawthorne Revisited*. Ithaca, NY: Cornell University Press, 1958; Sykes, A. J. M. 'Economics interests and the Hawthornes researches.' *Human Relations*, 18, 1965, pp. 253–63.

24 Re-analysis of Mayo's own data actually indicated that the 'friendliness' of the supervision . . . was probably as much an effect as a cause of increased productivity' and the greatest increases in productivity occurred in response to pay incentives. Ralph, *Work and Madness*. p. 77, citing Bramel, D., and Friend, R. 'Human relations in industry: The famous Hawthorne experiments.' Unpublished paper, State University of New York at Stony Brock, 1978.

25 Roethlisberger, F. J., and Dickson, W. J. *Management and the Worker: An Account of a Research Program Conducted by the Western Electric Company, Hawthorne Works, Chicago*. Cambridge, Mass.: Harvard University Press, 1939. p. 267.

26 Pavlov, Ivan. *Conditioned Reflexes: An Investigation of the Physiological Activity of the Cerebral Cortex*. New York: Dover Press. (Trans. G. V. Anrep, 1927.)

27 Watson, John B. *Behaviorism*. Chicago: University of Chicago Press, 1925. Revised 1930.

28 *Psychology from the Standpoint of a Behaviourist* (1919) explained how the principles of behaviour derived from animal studies could be applied to humans.

29 Reisman, J. *A History of Clinical Psychology*. New York: Irvington, 1976. p. 134.

30 Cushman, Philip. 'Psychotherapy to 1992: A historically situated interpretation.' In *History of Psychotherapy: A Century of Change*. Donald K. Freedheim (ed.) Washington, DC: American Psychological Association, 1992.

31 *Psychological Care of the Infant and Child* (1928) 'There is a sensible way of treating children: treat them as though they were young adults. Never hug or kiss them, never let them sit on your lap. If you must, kiss them once on the forehead when they say good-night. Shake hands with them in the morning. Let them learn to overcome difficulties from the moment of birth.'

32 R. M. Yerkes. 'Psychology in relation to the war.' In E. R. Hilgard (ed.) *American Psychology in Historical Perspective*. It is interesting to note that Yerkes, the American Psychological Association president at that time, was a major in the Sanitary Corp, as the Medical Corp was restricted to medical personnel only.

33 Lippmann, Walter. 'A future for the tests.' *New Republic*, 29 November 1922. p. 10.

34 Giberson, L. G. 'Industrial psychiatry: A wartime survey.' *The Medical Clinics of North America*, 26, 1942. p. 1088.

35 Industry began hiring psychiatrists as early as 1915 specifically to control 'grudge-bearers, agitators, drinkers, fighters and lazy persons' who threatened profits. Southward, E. E. 'The modern specialist in unrest: A place for the psychiatrist.' *Mental Hygiene*, 1920(A), 4, p. 557.

36 As Menninger (1963) noted, the history of psychiatry is largely a history of 'the urge to classify', an urge exemplified by his 70-page appendix of classification systems proposed in the interval from 2600 BC to AD 1959. Dineen. 'Diagnostic decision making in psychiatry.' p. 4.

37 Hutt, M. T., and Milton, E. O. 'An analysis of duties performed by clinical psychologists in the army.' *American Psychologist*, 2, 1947, pp. 52–56.

38 Kessen, W. 'The American child and other cultural inventions.' *American Psychologist*, 34(10), 1979, p. 820.

39 'Industrial and military influence dominated the formation of the NIMH, . . . and both business and government invested heavily in research to develop methods to treat large masses of people cheaply . . . Between 1948 and 1960, NIMH's budget increased almost 15-fold, from $4.5 million to $67.4 million.' Ralph. *Work and Madness*. pp. 96, 101.

40 Sarason. *Psychology Misdirected*. p. 34.

41 The writings of Skinner include *Walden Two*. New York: Macmillan, 1948; *Science and Human Behavior*. New York: Macmillan, 1953; *Beyond Freedom and Dignity*, New York: Alfred A. Knopf, 1971; *Cumulative Record: A Selection of Papers*. New York: Appleton-Century-Crofts, 1972; and *Reflections on Behaviorism and Society*. Engelwood Cliffs, NJ: Prentice-Hall, 1978.

42 The term 'black box' derives from physics, where it serves as a model of the functioning of any complex system. The black box is never considered to be empty; it is populated, often richly, with structures, constructs, operations and the like. Behaviourists, with an aversion to hypothesized internal mechanisms, misuse the original meaning of this term. (Reker, Arthur. *Dictionary of Psychology*. New York: Penguin, 1985.)

43 In 1957, the NIMH committed 8 per cent of its 'psychosocial' treatment research to behaviour modification, but by 1973 that share had grown to 55 per cent. Segal, J. (ed.) *Research in the Service of Mental Health*. Rockville, MD: National Institute of Mental Health, 1975. p. 329.

44 Such as Joseph Wolpe's *Psychotherapy by Reciprocal Inhibition* (1958) and Hans Eysenck's *Behaviour Therapy and the Neuroses* (1960).

45 London, Perry. *Behaviour Control* (2nd edn). New York: New American Library, 1977. p. 5.

46 Tennov, Dorothy. *Psychotherapy: The Hazardous Cure*. New York: Abelard-Schuman, 1975. p. 75. See also 'Psychotherapy as a means of social control' by Nathan Hurvitz (*Journal of Consulting and Clinical Psychology*, 40, 1973, pp.

232–39; *The Politics of Therapy* by Seymour L. Halleck (New York: Science House, 1971).

47 VandenBos, Gary R., Cummings, Nicholas A., and DeLeon, Patrick H. 'A century of psychotherapy: Economic and environmental influences.' In *History of Psychotherapy: A Century of Change.* p. 90.

48 Roszak, Theodore. *The Making of a Counter Culture; Reflections on the Technocratic Society and its Youthful Opposition.* Garden City, NY: Anchor Books, 1969. pp. xii–xiii.

49 Ibid. p. 233.

50 London, Perry. 'The psychotherapy boom: From the long couch for the sick to the push button for the bored.' *Psychology Today*, June 1974, pp. 63–68.

51 Ibid. p. 64.

52 Carkhuff, Robert R. *Helping and Human Relations: A Primer for Lay and Professional Helpers.* (Vols 1 and 2.) New York: Holt, Rinehart and Winston, 1969.

53 London. 'The psychotherapy boom.' p. 64.

54 Marathons originated with the work of George Bach and Frederick Stoller, and were shown to produce short-lived effects of good feelings.

55 Cited in London, Perry, and Klerman, Gerald L. 'Evaluating psychotherapy.' *American Journal of Psychiatry*, 139:6, June 1982 p. 709.

56 Herink, R. (ed) *The Psychotherapy Handbook: The A to Z Guide to More than 250 Different Therapies in Use Today.* New York: New American Library (Meridian), 1980.

57 VandenBos, Gary R., Cummings, Nicholas A., and DeLeon, Patrick H. 'A century of psychotherapy: Economic and environmental influences.' In Freedheim. *History of Psychotherapy.* p. 92.

58 Parloff, Morris B. 'Psychotherapy research evidence and reimbursement decisions: Bambi meets Godzilla.' *American Journal of Psychiatry*, 139(6), June 1982, p. 721.

59 Seligman, Martin E. P. 'Why therapy works.' *APA Monitor*, December 1998. p. 2.

60 'Landmark New Jersey lawsuit challenges no cause termination.' Practitioner Focus column by Cherie L. Jones, JD, and Shirley Ann Higuchi, JD. *APA Monitor*, August 1996.

61 Bickman, personal communication, 9 January 1999.

62 Strupp, Hans H., 'Is the medical model appropriate for psychoanalysis?' *Journal of the American Academy of Psychoanalysis*, 10(1). p. 124.

63 Chodoff, Paul. '*DSM-III* and Psychotherapy.' *American Journal of Psychiatry*, 143(2), 1986. pp. 201–3.

64 Dineen. 'Diagnostic Decision Making in Psychiatry.'
65 Cummings, Nicholas A. 'The anatomy of psychotherapy under national health insurance.' *American Psychologist*, September 1977, 711–21. p. 711.
66 Friedman, Matthew J., Charney, Dennis S., and Deutch, Ariel Y. 'Neurobiological and clinical consequences of stress: From normal adaptation to post-traumatic stress disorder.' Philadelphia: Lippincott-Raven, 1995.
67 Two relatively new medications, Naltrexone and Acamprosate, show promise for the treatment of patients with alcohol dependence, according to a new report on the effectiveness of medications used to treat alcoholism, developed by the North Carolina-based Research Triangle Institute and the University of North Carolina at Chapel Hill. 7 January 1999. PRNewswire.
68 The May 1996 issue of the *APA Monitor* addresses the 'active interest and controversy' of prescription privileges.
69 *Physicians Payment Review Commission: Annual Report to Congress 1989.* Washington, DC, 1990.
70 Gross. *The Psychological Society*. p. 4.
71 Parloff, M. B. 'Can psychotherapy research guide the policymaker? A little knowledge may be a dangerous thing.' *American Psychologist*, 34, 1979. pp. 296–306.
72 Thigpen, Corbett H., and Cleckley, Hervey M. 'On the incidence of multiple personality disorder: A brief communication.' *International Journal of Clinical and Experimental Hypnosis*, XXXII(2), 1984. pp. 63–66.
73 Putnam, Frank W. *Diagnosis and Treatment of Multiple Personality Disorder.* New York: Guilford Press, 1989. p. 47.
74 Borch-Jacobsen, Mikkel. 'Sybil – the making of a disease: An interview with Dr Herbert Spiegel.' *New York Review*, 24, 1997. p. 60.
75 For example, Rivera, Margo, *Multiple Personality: An Outcome of Child Abuse.* Toronto: Ontario Institute for Studies in Education, 1991; Ross, C. A., Norton, C. and Wozney, K. 'Multiple personality disorder: An analysis of 236 cases.' *Canadian Journal of Psychiatry*, 34(5), 1989. pp. 413–18.
76 The expectation (or demand) that patients accept the judgement of their doctors has been a primary standard of the profession for a long time. In 1888, the American Medical Association commanded patients to trust their doctors: 'The obedience of a patient to the prescriptions of his doctor should be prompt and implicit. The patient should never permit his own crude opinions as to their fitness to influence his attention to them.' *The Three Ethical Codes*. Detroit: Illustrated Medical Journal Co., 1888.
77 Raymond Fowler, chief executive officer of the APA in his 1994 Report. *American Psychologist*, August 1995. pp. 600–1.

78 Morris, Ted. 'CRHSPP Treasurer Dr. Ted Morris awarded OPA Award of Merit: "Calls colleagues to arms in face of growing Psychology 'crisis'".' *Rapport*, 3(1), 1995. p. 13.
79 Allon, Richard. 'And now for something completely different.' *Psynopsis*, Spring 1997. p. 4. Italics added.
80 Morris. As note 78.
81 For example, 'the National Conversation' of the American Psychological Association Practice Directorate, described in various places such as *Practitioner Update*, 3(2), 1995.
82 In a 1996 mail survey of nearly 1,000 mental-health care providers, 62 per cent of the responding psychologists reported earning less from their full-time practice than they did two years earlier. 'Practitioners report decrease in earnings.' *APA Monitor*, March 1997. p. 6.
83 Quoting Robert J. Resnick in 'New American Psychological Association president has keen vision for future' in *APA Monitor*, March 1995. p. 7.
84 Kovacs, A. 'The uncertain future of professional psychology.' *Independent Practitioner*, 9, 1989. pp. 11–18.
85 Herron, William G., and Welt, Sheila Rouslin. *Money Matters: The Fee in Psychotherapy and Psychoanalysis*. New York: Guilford Press, 1992. p. 168.
86 Therapist University: 'We train great therapists to be extraordinary coaches!' http://www.therapistu.com
87 'APA Public Education Campaign update.' *APA Monitor*, March 1997.
88 Wolf, Peter H. 'Psychoanalytic research and infantile sexuality.' *International Journal of Psychiatry*, 4(1), 1967. pp. 61–64.
89 Torrey, E. Fuller. *Witchdoctors and Psychiatrists*. New York: Harper & Row, 1986. p. 1.

Chapter 7

1 Noam Chomsky, personal communication, April 1998.
2 Ernest Becker. *The Denial of Death*. New York: Free Press, 1973.
3 Bollas, Christopher, and Sundelson, David. *The New Informant: The Betrayal of Confidentiality in Psychoanalysis and Psychotherapy*. Northvale, NJ: Jason Aronson, 1995. p. 105. 'Normopath', a defensive movement towards an extreme in normality, was created by Joyce McDougall (*A Plea for a Measure of Abnormality*. New York: International Universities Press, 1980) and 'Normotic' by Christopher Bollas (*The Shadow of the Object*. New York: Columbia University Press, 1987).

4 Smail. *Taking Care.* p. 142.

5 Niebuhr, Reinhold. *Beyond Tragedy: Essays on the Christian Interpretation of History.* North Stratford, NH: Ayer Co., 1977 (1938).

6 Langs, Robert. *Rating Your Psychotherapist: Everything You Need to Know to Find the Therapist Who's Right for You – From Getting Referrals to Ending Treatment.* New York: Ballantine Books, 1989, p. 5.

7 Hoffer, Eric. *The True Believer.* New York: Harper & Row, 1951. p. 118.

8 Smail. *Taking Care.* pp. 129–30.

9 Sarason, *Psychology Misguided.* p. 176.

10 Justice Brandeis, *Olmstead v. United States* 277 U.S. 438,479 (1928) (dissenting opinion).

11 Wiggins, Jack G., Jr. 'Would you want your child to be a psychologist?' *American Psychologist,* June 1994. p. 486.

12 Brandon, Sydney. 'Reported recovered memories of child sexual abuse.' *British Journal of Psychiatry,* April 1998. This followed the 1997 publication of consensus recommendations for good practice (Royal College of Psychiatrists Working Group on Reported Recovered Memories of Child Sexual Abuse, 1997).

13 Blackshaw, Stella, Chandarana, Praful, Garneau, Yvon, Merskey, Harold, and Moscarello, Rebeka. 'Adult recovered memories of childhood sexual abuse: Position statement.' *Canadian Journal of Psychiatry,* 41(5), 1996. pp. 305–6.

14 Prout, Phylis I., and Dobson, Keith. 'Middle Ground.' *Canadian Psychology,* 39(4), 1998. pp. 257–65.

15 Alec McGuire, chair of the British Association for Counselling, said the findings were unrepresentative. 'Brandon's report falls to one end of the spectrum. It does not express the consensus of the professions.' Cited by Rory Carroll in 'Recovered memory therapy is "useless".' *Guardian* (London), 1 April 1998. p. 4.

16 Franland, Alan, and Cohen, Lesley. 'Working with recovered memories.' *The Psychologist,* 12(2), 1999.

17 'World's psychology groups are burgeoning.' *APA Monitor,* 29(10), October 1998.

18 Marsella, Anthony J. 'Toward a "global-community psychology": Meeting the needs of a changing world.' *American Psychologist,* December 1998. pp. 1282–91.

19 Johnson, Robert A. *Owning Your Own Shadow.* San Francisco: Harper, 1991. pp. vii–viii.

20 May, Rollo. Foreword to Freedheim, *History of Psychotherapy.* pp. xx–xxvii.

21 Chambless, Dianne L., et al. 'Update on empirically validated therapies, II.' *Clinical Psychologist*, 51(1), 1998. pp. 3–16.
22 'The Barden Letter.' p. 3. Available from the National Association for Consumer Protection in Mental Health Practices, 937 Brunswick Circle, Schaumburg, IL. 60193, or at http://scholefieldhouse.com/mv/
23 Sarnoff, Susan. *Sanctified Snake Oil*. Wesport, CT: Praeger (in press).
24 An overview of the State version of the Truth and Responsibility in Mental Health Practices Act (draft 1/14/1995) p. 2. The state of Indiana has passed the informed consent portion of the Act (98–0 in the House and 58–0 in the Senate). The complete text and information about the legislation is available from the NACPMHP (see note 21).
25 For instance, 'finding a social mission,' Herman. *Trauma and Recovery*. p. 207 ff.
26 Brown, Laura S. 'The private practice of subversion: Psychology as Tikkum Olan.' *American Psychologist*, 52(4), April 1997. p. 453.
27 *Guardian Weekly*, 23 July 1995, 153(4), p. 9. In courts across the United States and Canada, lawsuits have begun to be heard.
28 *Humanne v. Humenansky* and *Carlson v. Humenansky*, 'Psychiatry in the courtroom.' *Law and Politics*, March 1996. pp. 34–39.
29 Zilbergeld, Bernie. The Shrinking of America: Myths of Psychological Change. Boston: Little, Brown & Co., 1983, p. 71.
30 Isaac, Rael Jean, and Arnat, Virginia C. *Madness in the Streets*. New York: Free Press, 1990; Torrey, E. Fuller. *Out of the Shadows: Confronting America's Mental Health Crisis*. New York: John Wiley, 1997.

Suggested Reading

Brown, E. Richard. *Rockefeller Medicine Men: Medicine and Capitalism in America.* Berkeley, CA: University of California Press, 1979.

Campbell, Terence W. *Beware the Talking Cure: Psychotherapy May Be Hazardous to Your Mental Health.* Boca Raton, FL: Upton Books, 1994.

Cecil, Stephen J., and Bruck, Maggie. *Jeopardy in the Courtroom: A Scientific Analysis of Children's Testimony.* Washington, DC: American Psychological Association, 1995.

Dantzer, Robert. *The Psychosomatic Delusion: Why the Mind Is Not the Source of All Our Ills.* New York: Free Press, 1993. (Originally published in French, 1989.)

Dawes, Robyn M. *House of Cards: Psychology and Psychotherapy Built on Myth.* New York: Macmillan, 1994.

Des Pres, Terrence. *The Survivor.* New York: Oxford University Press, 1976.

Eisner, Donald. *The Death of Psychotherapy: From Freud to Alien Abductions.* Westport, Connecticut: Greenwood Publishing Group (in press).

Fekete, John. *Moral Panic: Biopolitics Rising.* Montreal: Robert Davies, 1994.

Frank, J. D., and Frank, J. B. *Persuasion and Healing: A Comparative Study of Psychotherapy.* (3rd edn) Baltimore: Johns Hopkins University Press, 1991.

Freedheim, Donald K (ed.) *The History of Psychotherapy: A Century of Change.* Washington, DC: American Psychological Association, 1992.

Freyd, Pamela, and Goldstein, Eleanor. *Smiling Through Tears.* Boca Raton, FL: Upton Books, 1997.

Gist, R., and Lubin, B. *Response to Disaster: Psychosocial, Ecological and Community Approaches.* Philadelphia: Taylor & Francis (in press).

Goodyear-Smith, Felicity. *First Do No Harm: The Sexual Abuse Industry.* Auckland, New Zealand: Benton-Gay Publishing, 1993.

Gross, Martin L. *The Psychological Society: The Impact – and the Failure – of Psychiatry, Psychotherapy, Psychoanalysis and the Psychological Revolution.* New York: Random House, 1978.

Gross, Paul R., and Levitt, Norman. *Higher Superstition: The Academic Left and Its Quarrels with Science.* Baltimore: Johns Hopkins University Press, 1994.

Hacking, Ian. *Rewriting the Soul: Multiple Personality and the Sciences of Memory.* Princeton, NJ: Princeton University Press, 1995.

Hagen, Margaret A. *Whores of the Court: The Fraud of Psychiatric Testimony and the Rape of American Justice.* New York: Regan Books, HarperCollins, 1997.

Herman, Ellen. *The Romance of American Psychology: Political Culture in the Age of Experts.* Berkeley, CA: University of California Press, 1995.

Hillman, James, and Ventura, Michael. *We've Had a Hundred Years of Psychotherapy and the World Is Getting Worse.* San Francisco: HarperCollins, 1992.

Hoffer, Eric. *The True Believer.* New York: Harper & Row, 1951.

Huber, Peter W. *Galileo's Revenge: Junk Science in the Courtroom.* New York: HarperCollins, 1991.

Hughes, Robert. *The Culture of Complaint.* New York: Oxford University Press, 1993.

Kaminer, Wendy. *I'm Dysfunctional, You're Dysfunctional: The Recovery Movement and Other Self-Help Fashions.* New York: Vintage Books/Random House, 1993.

Lasch, Christopher. *Haven in a Heartless World: The Family Besieged.* New York: Basic Books, 1977.

Lasch, Christopher. *The Culture of Narcissism: American Life in an Age of Diminishing Expectations.* New York: W. W. Norton, 1979.

Loftus, E. F., and Ketcham, K. *The Myth of Repressed Memory.* New York: St Martin's Press, 1994.

May, Rollo. *Psychology and the Human Dilemma.* New York: W. W. Norton, 1967.

Nisbet, Robert. *History of the Idea of Progress.* New York: Basic Books, 1979.

Ofshe, Richard, and Watters, Ethan. *Making Monsters; False Memories, Psychotherapy, and Sexual Hysteria.* New York: Charles Scribner's Sons, 1994.

Oppenheim, Janet. *'Shattered Nerves'. Doctors, Patients, and Depression in Victorian England.* Oxford: Oxford University Press, 1991.

Peele, Stanton. *Diseasing of America: Addiction Treatment Out of Control.* Lexington, Mass.: Lexington Books, 1989.

Pious, Scott. *The Psychology of Judgement and Decision-Making.* New York: McGraw, 1993.

Pendergrast, Mark. *Victims of Memory: Incest Accusations and Shattered Lives.* London: HarperCollins, 1997.

Ralph, Diana. *Work and Madness: The Rise of Community Psychiatry.* Montreal: Black Rose Books, 1983.

Revel, Jean-François. *The Flight from Truth.* New York: Random House, 1991.

Roiphe, Katie. *The Morning After: Sex, Fear and Feminism on Campus.* Boston: Little, Brown, 1993.

Sarason, Seymour B. *Psychology Misdirected.* New York: Free Press, 1981.

Sarnoff, Susan Kiss. *Sanctified Snake Oil.* Westport, CT: Praeger Publishers, in press.

Schultz, Duane P. *A History of Modern Psychology.* New York: Academic Press, 1969.

Showalter, Elaine. *Hystories: Hysterical Epidemics and Modern Media.* New York: Columbia University Press, 1997.

Smail, David. *Taking Care: An Alternative to Therapy.* London: J. M. Dent & Sons, 1987.

Smail, David. *How to Survive Without Psychotherapy.* London: Constable, 1996.

Smith, Susan. *Survivor Psychology: The Dark Side of a Mental Health Mission.* Boca Raton, FL: Upton Books, 1995.

Sykes, Charles J. *A Nation of Victims: The Decay of the American Character.* New York: St Martin's Press, 1992.

Sykes, Charles. *Dumbing Down Our Kids: Why American Children Feel Good About Themselves but Can't Read, Write or Add.* New York: St Martin's Press, 1995.

Szasz, Thomas. *The Myth of Psychotherapy: Mental Healing as Religion, Rhetoric, and Repression.* Garden City, NY: Anchor Press/Doubleday, 1978.

Szasz, Thomas. *The Manufacture of Madness: A Comparative Study of the Inquisition and the Mental Health Movement.* New York: Harper & Row, 1970.

Tennov, Dorothy. *Psychotherapy: The Hazardous Cure.* New York: Abelard-Schuman, 1975.

Torrey, E. Fuller. *Witchdoctors and Psychiatrists.* New York: Harper & Row, 1986 (revised and reprinted as *The Mind Game: Witchdoctors and Psychiatrists.* New York: Aronson, 1994).

Torrey, E. Fuller. *Freudian Fraud: The Malignant Effect of Freud's Theory on American Thought and Culture.* New York: HarperCollins, 1993.

Zilbergeld, Bernie. *The Shrinking of America: Myths of Psychological Change.* Boston: Little, Brown, 1983.

Ziskin, Jay. *Coping with Psychiatric and Psychological Testimony.* (Volumes 1–5) Los Angeles: Law and Psychology Press, 1995.

Index

Printed in the United Kingdom by
Lightning Source UK Ltd., Milton Keynes
142053UK00001B/45/A

9 780094 797901